D1482379

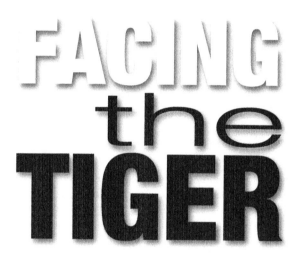

FACING the TIGER

A Guide for Men with Prostate Cancer
and the People Who Love Them

Professor Suzanne Chambers
Psychologist

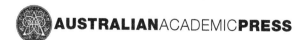
AUSTRALIANACADEMIC**PRESS**

First published in January 2013 by Australian Academic Press Group Pty. Ltd.
Level 5, Toowong Tower, 9 Sherwood Road,
Toowong QLD 4066, Australia
www.australianacademicpress.com.au

National Library of Australia Cataloguing-in-Publication entry:

Author:	Chambers, Suzanne.
Title:	Facing the tiger : a guide for men with prostate cancer and the people who love them / Suzanne Chambers.
ISBN:	9781922117052 (pbk.)
Subjects:	Prostate--Cancer--Popular works.
	Prostate--Diseases--Patients--Popular works.
	Cancer--Patients--Family relationships
	Cancer--Patients--Long-term care.

Dewey Number: 616.994

DISCLAIMER: Every effort has been made in preparing this work to provide information based on accepted evidence, standards and practice at the time of publication. By referring to this book, any and all readers release the author and publisher of any claims of direct or consequential damages resulting from relying on the content contained herein.

Book and cover design by Maria Biaggini — The Letter Tree.
Image by ©istockphoto/Dirk Freder

'Suzanne Chambers is one of those rare people who not only sees a problem but immediately starts to think about how to do something about it. So much of the psycho-oncology literature is full of studies about observation and measurement. Suzanne's group is leading the way in devising meaningful interventions based on this knowledge and then testing whether they actually make a difference. Suzanne has taken her practical insights and loaded them into this easy-to-read book, illustrating them with real examples. This book will make a large difference to the lives of people affected by prostate cancer.'

— Professor Ian Davis, Medical Oncologist, Founder and Chair, Australian and New Zealand Urogenital and Prostate Cancer Trials Group

'Suzanne Chambers has written the game plan for coping with prostate cancer. She brings years of experience from observing how men and their mates cope. She also presents the "how to" in terms that are understandable and acceptable. Football is a great metaphor for successful coping: working closely with the coach/oncologist; taking the offensive and charging forward; maintaining optimism and confidence; keeping an eye on the goal despite transient setbacks; being sure the whole team is working together. The stories in the book show how courage pays off, how engaging the spouse helps both in coping, and how humour and empathy ease the bruises of the game. It is a MUST for those coping with this type of cancer.'

— *Professor Jimmie Holland, MD. Wayne E. Chapman Chair in Psychiatric Oncology, Attending Psychiatrist, Department of Psychiatry & Behavioral Sciences, Memorial Sloan-Kettering Cancer Center, New York*

'An excellent hand-book. Suzanne Chambers has had an enduring and innovative commitment to helping to resolve the many difficulties encountered by those involved with prostate cancer for many years. Tracing the many dilemmas faced in what is so often a long journey with this condition, this book proposes practical ways to straddle the hurdles that appear in the paths of patients and partners. The book is written 'from the heart' and provides a self-help guide in simple and unambiguous language. A major strength is the inclusion of sections by a number of courageous patients and partners who have openly shared what are so often regarded as private experiences.'

— *Professor RA ('Frank') Gardiner AM, MBBS MD FRACS FRCS, Professor of Urology, The University of Queensland, Consultant Urologist, Royal Brisbane & Women's Hospital*

'A must-read for all patients, and their families, who are faced with a diagnosis of prostate cancer and the life after it. The medical community is still in the infancy of incorporating issues of patient distress and the psycho-social elements of therapeutic care into clinical practice. This book helps medical consumers find their internal strength and empowers them to be advocates for their own best quality of life.'

— Virgil H. Simons, MPA, Founder & President,
The Prostate Net, an international non-profit patient education
and advocacy organization for men with prostate cancer

'Once a patient, partner/carer or a family member affected by prostate cancer starts to read this book they will not be able to put it down. It is a wonderful blend of real life stories, practical tips learnt by experience and professional know how. Quality of life is a theme that resonates along with confidence building and knowing you are not alone.'

— David Sandoe OAM, National Chairman Prostate Cancer
Foundation of Australia and co-leader (with his wife Pam) of the
Sydney Adventist Hospital Prostate Cancer Support Group

'A must read for anybody coping with a prostate cancer diagnosis. It is equally as useful and important for their partners. I wish it had been around when I was diagnosed.'

— Peter Dornan AM, Sport Physiotherapist, Author, Sculptor and
Convenor of the Brisbane Prostate Cancer Support Network

Contents

Acknowledgments

I have been privileged over many years to have had
men affected by prostate cancer and their loved ones
share their often very difficult experiences with me.
This book has grown out of those shared experiences.
A heart felt thank you to David and Pam Sandoe for
suggesting that I write this book and encouraging me
at every step, and to my trusted friend and colleague,
clinical psychologist Samantha Clutton for reading
every chapter and giving me fearless feedback! To Jeff
Dunn, my long standing friend and colleague, I appreciate you reminding me to make a point, and a difference. I thank Ysabella Chambers, my daughter, who is
herself a writer, for editorial advice and guidance on
speaking with a true voice. Many other colleagues,
Leslie Schover, Rob Newton, David Jenkins, and
Daniel Galvao, also provided expert advice for which
I am so grateful, and I thank Anthony Lowe and
Prostate Cancer Foundation of Australia for their
support of this book. To my urological and medical

colleagues, thank you for trusting me with your patients, and for teaching me the difference between a pussy cat and a tiger.

Finally, my deepest thanks to all the men and women, many of whom I am fortunate to count as friends, who so generously shared their personal stories in this book.

■■■■

Foreword

Footballers understand the old saying that 'no man is an island'. We know that the key to advantage in football is a strong team, a good game plan, and the ability to collectively cope with unforeseen incursions from the opposing side.

The key to coping with prostate cancer is similar. And yet oddly, for many of us, a diagnosis of prostate cancer sidelines us from our partners, our family and our friends.

Facing the Tiger is mandatory reading for all men seeking a game plan for dealing with prostate cancer, and for the people who care most about them. It provides down-to-earth advice on understanding the challenges and defending against them, with stories of hope and optimism from ordinary Australians who have tackled the disease.

The author, Suzanne Chambers (Professor to those who don't know her), has over twenty years of experience in the field. She has seen firsthand what men and their partners go through, and has developed practical and well-tried strategies that you can easily put into play.

This book will help you find the courage to face the tiger. The next step is up to you.

Ron Coote AM
Founder and National President
Men of League

■■■■

Facing the Tiger

Being told you have prostate cancer is for most men, and those close to them, an experience they will never forget. At that moment, the world seems changed. The things that you may have taken for granted are now at threat. While health care professionals and others around you may honestly express their concern and sympathy, this can be a singularly lonely and distressing time.

You are not alone. Prostate cancer is now the most common male cancer in the western world, excluding non-melanoma skin cancer. The most recent estimates are that in the United States over 2.5 million men are living with a diagnosis of prostate cancer; in the United Kingdom over 250,000 men, and in Australia over 120,000 men. The incidence of prostate cancer in Asia is less well documented but growing. For each man who has had prostate cancer, there will be people close who care about them, and love them, who are also deeply affected. This book is for you too.

The aim of this book is to provide a map to help you see a way through this difficulty and find a path that helps you to regain a sense of ease about the situation in which you have found yourself, and the way the world looks to you now. This is not a guide book about treatment options and will not give any medical advice. We list places where you can find this type of advice at the end of the book in an appendix and your doctor who knows your medical circumstances is always your first port of call.

This book is about suggesting different perspectives on where you are now, where you would like to be as you move forward in your cancer journey, and proven strategies that might help you get there. You may even find these techniques helpful in other aspects of your life and should feel free to apply them if you think they seem to be relevant. The book is structured so that each chapter works on its own and you can choose what part seems most relevant to you now. It includes personal stories from different men and women who have been in the same situation as you and we hope you will find this both comforting and inspiring. Everyone's experience of prostate cancer is their own, and there is no one right or wrong way to approach this. However, there is nothing quite like personal experience and the wisdom that comes from this experience.

Why do I feel like this?

A common way to explain why the experience of cancer causes feelings of anxiety or sadness, is to describe it as a *major life stress*. A major life stress is when an event happens to us that causes threat or danger to things that matter to us most. Cancer is a threat that goes to the core of us. It is first and foremost a threat to life and survival, and many people report that the first question they asked their doctor after hearing the news was: 'Will this cancer kill me?'

Cancer can also be a threat to a person's sense of self: 'Will I be the same as I was before or will I be changed? Less me in some way? Will I still be able to do the things that matter to me?' Cancer can threaten a person's relationships: 'Will I still be loved and cared for? Will people want to be close to me?'

So, no surprises then, that a diagnosis of cancer is often (almost always) accompanied by feelings of fear, shock ('I never heard a word after I heard him say it was cancer!'), anger, deep sadness and confusion. You might have found it hard to concentrate, and had physical signs of stress such as an upset stomach, feeling on edge or irritable, or had restless sleep. Perhaps you find yourself still feeling this way, some or a lot of the time.

A way of explaining why this happens is to think of what would happen if you were facing a tiger! We are all organisms made to recognise threats and respond in a way that will protect ourselves from harm. So, if you were a hunter (or a gatherer) and you found yourself faced by a tiger, your body would instantly recognise the tiger as a serious threat to life and well-being, and would get you ready biologically to fight or to run (the 'fight or flight' response). Your body does this through an immediate hormonal reaction where your adrenal glands (on top of your kidneys) pump out adrenalin and noradrenalin, and these internal chemicals make your heart go faster, your mouth feel dry, your pupils dilate, and your gut stop working (among a few other things), you become poised to respond to the tiger in front of you. And while that's all quite helpful in the face of an actual tiger, its not so helpful when the threat is cancer! Instead, right when you are thinking about and trying to rationally work out what the cancer diagnosis means for you, your body is sending out physical fear reactions, and the emotions that go with this are inevitably unpleasant, such as feeling sad, anxious, or afraid.

The very good news is that you can do something about this. There are skills and strategies you can learn to help you meet the problems cancer brings and better manage both physical and emotional challenges. That is what this book is about, explaining ways to moderate or manage psychological and coping responses to cancer, in order to live your life fully, the way that you wish.

An important point to make here is that cancer is not just one experience. It is a journey marked by different hurdles. The first hurdle is the diagnosis itself, learning about the extent and nature of the cancer and what treatment options are possible. As a time of uncertainty and distress this one heads the list. Once a decision about treatment is made a feeling of calm may come, at least until the preparation for and time of treatment, and then it is 'action stations' again. Recovering from treatment can also be tough, especially learning how to manage any treatment side effects, such as urinary continence, erectile dysfunction, or bowel problems. Medical checkups can be stressful, especially PSA test time (sometimes unhelpfully called PSA-itis). In the longer term, the issue that many men and their partners find most challenging is coping with sexual changes. Our sexual self is a big part of who we are and an important part of many relationships, so changes in this area can be devastating. Acknowledging the aspects of prostate cancer that are most hard and the loss and changes prostate cancer may have brought to your life is part of healing, and allows you to make choices about how to move forward.

How do I move forward?

As you progress though this book you will be asked to reflect on your experiences, your strengths, what works well for you, and some of the ways you might not serve yourself well. We want you to become your own best friend. A journal or notebook to jot down your thoughts and reflections will help you in this process, and will mark the changes as you go along.

You will also see in each chapter an Activity section with practical questions and tasks for you to do. These are based on my experiences of working with men and their partners from all sorts of backgrounds. They can be very helpful to your journey in dealing with cancer and I strongly recommend that you take the time when ready to read and undertake these activities.

Activity

As a first step think about how you felt when you first found out about the cancer and see if you can recall the thoughts that ran through your mind. Did you have one strong worry, or a stream of concerns that rapidly replaced each other? Was there one strong emotion you felt? How did your body respond physically? What was your first coping reaction? Did you look for a cave for comfort or did you come out fighting?

Draw a map on a piece of paper with four circles, one for thoughts, one for emotions, one for physical reactions and one for actions. Now fill in examples in each box of what sort of thoughts, emotions, physical reactions and actions you remember feeling and doing. What actions did you take that were helpful? What did not work so well? Now think back to a different example in your life when you have had a difficult time, perhaps a job loss, serious illness in someone you cared for, the death of a loved one, the end of a relationship. Were your feelings then similar to now, or different? Do you have a typical way of coping with stress, and how well does this serve you?

Personal Stories

Reading personal stories from others can help you to reflect more deeply on your own experience; can give you new ideas about how to manage difficulties as they arise; inspire you about what is possible after cancer; and help you feel less alone in your experience. You might like to think about how these stories are similar or different to your personal story. Remember everyone is different and there is no one single right or wrong way to cope. Below are personal stories from husband and wife David and Pam about their experiences with prostate cancer, the challenges they faced, and how they overcame these.

David

I was working at Zurich Financial Services when I went along for the usual executive health check. Following the full check up, which included a PSA blood test and a digital rectal examination (DRE), I was told to see a urologist immediately. He performed a biopsy and confirmed I had cancer.

For anyone to be told this, it's a big shock. One of the dilemmas for me was whether to be open with my staff and friends. I'm open, by nature, so I went back to the office and with a bit of difficulty told the people closest to me the verdict. The next weekend I informed my closest friends. That sent shockwaves through people of my own age group. I was 51 then. Many friends and colleagues of my age underwent similar tests and one of them was in hospital weeks later for heart bypass surgery.

Treatment options for prostate cancer depend on your age and the severity of the cancer. Because I was relatively young, 50 years old, and had no symptoms, a radical prostatectomy was a real option for me as the urologist was confident I had a cancer that was confined to the prostate.

Treatment options for prostate cancer can result in incontinence and impotence. The medical professionals try for the trifecta: to get rid of the cancer and have good continence and erectile function. After surgery I was incontinent for a while. That was soon overcome with pelvic floor exercises but the operation rendered me impotent. Over the years erectile function did come back but not enough for penetration so my wife Pam and I have had to try other methods. Initially I tried oral medications — that didn't work and then injection therapy but suffered great pain with a chemical reaction. The vacuum device was our next option and our relationship and sex life was as good as it had ever been. However, it was a tedious process at first. Six and a half years ago I put my reluctance for another operation to one side and had a penile prosthesis implanted. I can now faithfully report that after 45 years of marriage our 'love making' could not be better.

I'm now in my sixteenth year since my radical prostatectomy. I do realise someday the cancer may come back and I'm prepared for that. Prostate cancer is something I wouldn't wish on my worst enemy but having been through the experience Pam and I now appreciate life to the fullest extent. Family, friends and my business network are all very important to me and I work hard to maximise my opportunities, endeavouring to make a difference every day. These days I'm working hard on raising awareness and making it easier for those diagnosed with Prostate Cancer, their carers and family. I'm National Chairman of Prostate Cancer Foundation of Australia (PCFA) and together with Pam, we lead the Sydney Adventist Hospital — Prostate Cancer Support Group. PCFA now has affiliated Prostate Cancer Support Groups across Australia in every state and territory. I'm an advocate for regular checks and talking to your doctor about men's health generally, especially for those 50 or over. Us blokes need to wake-up and take our health seriously.

You would not wish prostate cancer on your worst enemy, but the challenging experience Pam and I faced as a loving couple has enriched our lives.

Pam

Just hearing the word 'cancer' means emotional turmoil. We were no different. Like a lot of men, David thought himself fairly bullet proof, and it was with some reluctance and the insistence of the CEO of Zurich Financial Services, that all the executives underwent a full medical check. David was the first to report a problem! When he announced the results the news sent shock waves amongst his colleagues and friends in the insurance industry. Our family and friends were also stunned.

David had no idea if there was any family medical history that could have rung alarm bells previously.

After a long consult with our urologist that confirmed cancer we left his rooms trying to make sense of how, why and what next needed to be done to get our thought processes working properly and how to best 'attack' what lay ahead. David is of the opinion that most things can be overcome and life can be made easier by being well organised. We elected to start by making yet another long list.

This included questions for our GP, a consult with a Radiation Oncologist and foremost, letting our teenage children know of the outcome. The burning question of 'who do you tell', beyond immediate family, and should work colleagues be included, was quickly decided as David is a very open person. We were upfront and let everyone know.

The list of those important items to be looked at included attending to financial papers, our wills, and David's work situation. We weren't surprised when some people found it difficult and uncomfortable to talk over the diagnosis with us.

Coping with the cancer diagnosis included wondering what the end result would be and learning more about the prostate and its function. Do we really need it? Can we live without it? How will the treatment affect our relationship?

We quickly learnt that only about 10% of what the medical professional is telling you will sink in. Hopefully that person (and other consultants) will give you some written information to take away, whether it is notes used in describing your biopsy results or more importantly, diagrams of your anatomy with informative booklets and leaflets on the subject. We certainly found it of great benefit to both be included in the consultations. Two sets of ears mean you'll remember more. After all, if you are in a relationship, it is very much a couples issue.

The emotional turmoil includes anger, denial, confusion and frustration. Here we were at 50 and 51, 'in the prime of our lives' and we are confronted with cancer which we thought was 'an old man's disease'. Before all this happened we did not even know how to pronounce 'prostate' cancer let alone understand that the implications were. What a learning curve!

It was important to understand the treatment options available but as some of the newer options weren't around, ours included doing nothing (watchful waiting as it was then called),a radical prostatectomy (surgery), or external beam radiation therapy. In David's case, all agreed that surgery was his best bet of ridding himself of the cancer and David still states that if he had his time over he'd proceed with this choice. And I agree. It's of little benefit to suddenly have tunnel vision whether you're the patient or the carer. Communication during this time is paramount. Women share personal experiences with other women. We ask questions, seek information and manage health issues and are proactive in undergoing tests. We want men to become the same. Our close friends rallied to discuss the choices, read up on the disease, understand our situation and gave us the added confidence that we were making the right choice. It helped that one of these friends has a long history with breast cancer.

Thankfully too, our urologist had a great 'game plan' in that he used his patients to telephone counsel newly diagnosed men. What a relief to have the lovely voice of a fellow patient speaking to David and to give him confidence about the road ahead. Friends and colleagues who had undergone this type of surgery soon rallied when they heard the news. It was a 'security blanket' we couldn't have done without as any little hitch in the process of recovery was dealt with by a simple phone call.

David was a great patient, which I was surprised about! His recovery went according to plan. Each day was different — emotions soared, rest and recuperation was well monitored and on occasions visitors and phone calls restricted by me. We appreciated everyone's concerns. By the time he was ready to return to the office he'd overcome his incontinence with pelvic floor exercises but the ongoing issue of erectile dysfunction was another learning curve.

As a seasoned carer of parents and elderly relatives, I made sure I was eating well, taking time out and getting some exercise — probably not enough, but under the circumstances, apart from the emotional rollercoaster I survived. Communicating with those nearest and dearest to me gave me the ultimate support I needed!

■ ■ ■ ■

'Why me?'
On Being Diagnosed
With Prostate Cancer

Before going any further it is important to remember that individuals differ. This seems like a simple statement that we all know and agree with, but we often operate in the world as if everyone thinks and acts like we do, and if they don't they should. While some people may react to life a lot like you, mostly they won't, and this includes people close to you. Accepting this upfront can help prevent misunderstanding. Accepting your own reaction to being diagnosed with prostate cancer as just that — your own — is crucial. In other words, guard against judging yourself (or others) and give yourself a break!

The things that influence how a person reacts to a cancer diagnosis include age, gender, educational background, and previous life experiences. We know this from relentless research in the field, however it just makes sense if you think it through. For example, younger men often report higher levels of distress than older men, and this may relate to the stage of life younger men are at, perhaps still raising children, building a career, not being financially well established and certainly not expecting a cancer diagnosis at this age. Some younger men with prostate cancer may not yet have had children, or are hoping for more children, and so face the potential loss of fertility. Perhaps their intimate relationship is new and not yet well established, or they do not have a partner and fear that now it will be even harder to form a relationship.

For older men the issues may be different. Older men may finally have retired from the full time workforce and be gearing up to enjoy a different pace of life and to doing the things they have long dreamed about, like a 'grey nomad' holiday, playing more golf, or spending time with grandchildren. Older men may be facing other health problems as well, such as heart disease or arthritis, and these things can make it harder to manage the physical problems associated with prostate cancer and its treatment.

What does cancer mean to me?

Previous personal experience with cancer also has an impact on how a man reacts to a cancer diagnosis. A man has a higher chance of being diagnosed with prostate cancer if he has a first degree relative (a father or brother) who has had prostate cancer. If your relative had a difficult time with prostate cancer and perhaps did not do well after treatment, this will influence your expectations and fears about what might happen to you. Beyond this, as we age it is almost impossible not to have friends or relatives with cancer given that older age is a risk factor for the most common cancers such as breast, colorectal and prostate cancer. Whatever the nature of the cancer experiences we have observed, we can't help but weave this into our internal or mental picture of what having cancer means. If you have known people who managed well after cancer you may see your prostate cancer as a challenge that you can overcome. However, if your personal experiences of cancer have been mostly negative your prostate cancer may seem like a huge looming threat.

Why does this matter? Having cancer can feel overwhelming and confusing. If you can gain some understanding of what lies underneath or directs your strongest reactions you will be better able to manage your response in a way that works more effectively for you. For example, if you are clear about which of your life goals are most threatened by the cancer, you can direct efforts to plan how you might still achieve those goals, but in a different way. If you had a very negative personal cancer experience in the past that is influencing how you are responding now, you can challenge the actual relevance of this past experience to your current situation. Getting clear about your life goals and what cancer means to you is important in making sense of where you are right now.

Being a Man and Coping with Cancer

What also matters is understanding your own personal coping style. Most of us have our own typical approaches to problems or challenges. A lot of this is learnt in our childhood by what our parents and our peer group tells us, and what they model by their own behaviour. It is fair to say that boys are taught or expected to be strong and fearless. If you break this approach down to what it means in terms of behaviour, you could reasonably list: don't cry when you are hurt; keep your feelings to yourself; take risks; fight back; be self-reliant; and if it is broken, just fix it! These strategies are often described as male stoicism: the 'hang tough' and 'be a man' approach — recognise any of this? As a result, compared to women, men seek preventative health care services less often; are less likely to report depression but more likely to commit suicide; and are much less likely to use cancer support services. In brief, many blokes approach their health in ways that are just not that helpful; that make it tougher for themselves in the short and long term; and that to their detriment bottle up difficult emotions and block support.

A disclaimer however — I am not suggesting you need to change your personality! The key is to decide, in the face of a prostate cancer diagnosis, to adopt strategies that help you rather than hinder you. A helpful analogy here is to think about coping strategies as tools in your toolbox. You would not try to change a tyre using an everyday shifting spanner or wrench unless you wanted to make things really hard for yourself. When you work on a car you have a box full of tools where each tool works differently for different parts of the engine and chassis. In coping with cancer you might have one tool you prefer the most, but if it doesn't seem to be working or getting you the results you want, then another tool might make things a lot easier.

Coping approaches or tools are often put into two broad groups: problem solving or emotion focussed. *Problem solving coping* is just that — applying strategies to solve the problem. The aim is to fix it. In the case of a prostate cancer diagnosis this might mean seeking different medical opinions, looking up medical information on the Internet, making a decision, and having treatment. Problem solving is an active approach that achieves outcomes and helps you to move forward in a practical and tangible way.

Emotion focussed coping applies strategies to reduce painful or difficult emotions or feelings of distress. This can include talking to other people about how you feel, crying or expressing emotion, and using stress management and relaxation techniques. These strategies are useful in keeping an even keel and managing how you feel while going through the cancer, and are a natural complement to problem solving.

Avoiding thinking (or talking) about the cancer is another type of emotion focussed coping that can be helpful in some situations, and not so helpful in others. For example, if you are about to have a biopsy or a painful medical procedure, not thinking about this and instead imagining you are on a beach in Fiji might be very helpful as a short-term distraction. However, imagining you are in Fiji all or most of the time will likely hinder your ability to make decisions and communicate with others close to you about what is happening in your life.

The trick then is to use flexible coping, being prepared to change tack if your current approach is not working and being open to possibilities and change. In brief, you want a tool box that will help you get the best outcome you can for yourself and for those close to you.

What are the likely issues I will face in the future?

Over time, most men find that the difficult feelings they experience when they are diagnosed ease. Life starts to return to normal (although many say a 'different normal') and unless a specific issue comes up, like a PSA blood test or a health complication, they feel life is just as good as it was before the cancer. The most persistent long-term problem for men is usually on the sexual side of things. Most prostate cancer treatments lead to changes in sexual function, for example, being unable to get an erection or an erection not as firm as before treatment, and a loss of sexual desire. For men this can have a deep effect on how they see themselves as a man. Many men have told me they feel less vital as a result of these sexual changes and that getting themselves back to feeling masculine and confident with sex and relationships has been difficult, and for many is still a 'work in progress'.

Other worries can include ongoing tiredness, and this may be a result of treatment or of the stress associated with the whole cancer experience. Tiredness can make it difficult to get back to usual activities and the things that you enjoy. While treatment effects on urinary and bowel function often resolve in the short- to medium-term, coping with these in the meantime requires planning and effort. If a man is having hormone blocking treatment this can lead to tiredness, a low mood, loss of muscle strength and poorer mental concentration. Strategies to maintain well-being are crucial.

For many men a feeling of uncertainty about the future and whether the cancer will come back is an ongoing worry. Regardless of the fact that one day we will all die (that is for certain), most of us live as if our days ahead are endless. A diagnosis of cancer means that dying of cancer is a possibility (although again this is actually true for all of us), and it forces most people to, at least at some level, contemplate their mortality. In this sense the world can appear very different after a diagnosis of prostate cancer — less fair or just — and coming to terms with and accepting a changed under-standing of the world and our place in it is a journey all of its own.

Setting Goals

One thing is for sure, if you don't know where you want to go, you probably won't get there! Setting goals is crucial to the approach we suggest in this book. Goals can be short, medium and long term. The trick is for them to be realistic, achievable, important to you, and that you are able to tell when you have got there. A 'small steps' first approach is usually best here.

Activity

For all men at whatever stage of life, prostate cancer threatens their goals and hopes. How has cancer affected your goals and future hopes? Write these down in your notebook. Perhaps your goals have changed since the cancer diagnosis and other things have become more important. Looking at your list, which of these matter most you right now?

Each of your goals will have a different timeline, some might be things you would like to achieve in the short- or medium-term, some might be long-term goals. You might set goals that are about how you are coping with the cancer; or about your relationships and how you would like them to be or to develop. As an example, a short-term goal might be to learn some quick and easy stress reduction strategies, such as deep breathing exercises and a low intensity walking program. As you do this you can map your overall wellbeing so you can be encouraged by the gains you make. A plan to improve your sexual life might start with short-term goals about pleasant couple activities (such as seeing a movie or going for a dinner 'date') and intimacy, and sensual pleasure, with a medium-term goal to have full sexual intercourse. Long-term goals might be to complete treatment and then go on a long awaited holiday (best not to wait for 'one day') or to take on a personal physical or mental challenge. You might have long-term life goals you would like to work towards.

What would you like life to look like for you in six or twelve months' time?

Next, start to list what steps that you need to take to achieve these goals? Finally, who can help you with this? Jot down the names of people in your life you could enlist to support, help or encourage you to reach these goals. Talk to someone you trust or who is close to you about your most hoped for goals. This will help you further clarify and confirm your next steps. Every month or so check back with your list and see how you are going. It is perfectly fine if your list changes, or if new goals come up. The main point of this activity is that you have a sense of direction and that you notice when you achieve goals, and then give yourself a pat on the back!

Now for your tool box! How do you usually cope with difficulties? What is your main preference and how well does that work for you? Think about a time when you have coped well with a personal challenge and felt very positive about the outcome. How would you describe your approach then? Now think about a time when you were faced with a personal challenge and it did not go so well. How could you have approached this problem differently?

Further on in this book you will find more specific suggestions and ideas about ways to face prostate cancer and to tame the tiger! Feel free to jump ahead, but you might find it helps to do the reflections suggested in this chapter in advance and prioritise your goals.

Personal Stories

Below is a personal story from Peter about his experience with prostate cancer at a young age, the difficulties he faced after surgery, and the strategies he used to move forward. Your experience may be similar in some ways to Peters' story, or very different. A fairly common element though that men do report is feeling you are alone, and as Peter's story shows, this need not be the case.

Peter

When I was diagnosed with prostate cancer at the age of 52, (in 1996), after a routine blood test (PSA), the shock was enormous. At the time, such was the neglected state of awareness of men's health issues, I didn't even know what my prostate was — or, for that matter, what it did. As well, as a health professional — a physiotherapist — for the previous twenty years I had followed a lifestyle of exercise, diet and meditation, one which the gurus had promised would significantly lessen the risk of cardiac disease and cancer. Not completely true, I found.

To add to the shock, virtually any invasive treatment I could undertake had the potential of being nasty. To me, at the time, surgery (radical prostatectomy) seemed to offer the best chance for survival. At this stage, some sixteen years later, it certainly appears to have achieved that — something for which I am decidedly grateful.

However, after the prostatectomy in February 1996, I was left severely incontinent, to the extent where I was filling six incontinence pads a day during the first six months. I found that this was seriously impacting on my lifestyle, as well as my professional career, emotional health, exercise activity, sex life and relationships. In fact, I was also suffering from erectile dysfunction, a situation in itself I was not coping with. I became very despondent and developed reactive depression. Worse still, I could find no other men who had been through this process. I felt very isolated. In my mind, I was the only man in the world in this situation.

The frustration, anger — and indeed, often rage — I felt led me to resolve to change things. The alternative was to accept a seriously reduced lifestyle. In fact, suicide appeared an attractive proposition. The vulnerable time was driving home from work — tired, leaking and devastated that love making may never by a reality again. I really was feeling hopeless and despairing.

It was then that a quiet voice deep inside took command and ordered me to quell my panic — to be calm. In desperation, I sought out some physiotherapy colleagues who I knew treated women with incontinence. They taught me how to execute standard pelvic floor muscles exercises, which I performed aggressively and with enormous motivation. The action began to stem the flow and after some months, I had controlled the loss to about a dozen leakages a day. While this was more acceptable and manageable in terms of my lifestyle, I still found that just one leakage would trigger a depression cycle, one of the now obvious psycho-social legacies resulting from my choice of treatment.

At this stage, I put an advertisement in the local paper and formed the first Prostate Cancer Support Group in Queensland. From this, I hoped to find some answers to assist both me and the many others I soon found who were fellow sufferers. (With the assistance of Cancer Council Queensland, the Brisbane Prostate Cancer Support Group is now one of the largest groups in the country, and we have joined with other groups nationally as part of Prostate Cancer Foundation of Australia. No man need be alone again!)

I then worked to improve my incontinence to another level. Some four years after diagnosis, I designed an intensive exercise program aiming to develop a highly efficient (super fit) neuromuscular and vascular system which controls and supplies all the structures that form the pelvic and abdominal cavities. The idea was to increase the local and collateral pelvic circulation. For me, that meant endurance type exercise — running, cycling, and gym. As well, I wanted to retrain elements of the neural reflex circuitry of all the muscles and sphincters which control continence. I did this with jogging, firstly on flat ground, then uneven ground, then uphills, harder and faster. Finally, I worked on integrating pelvic floor muscle activity with abdominal muscle activity. This meant contracting the pelvic floor muscles and the abdominal muscles simultaneously while functionally doing 'crunches'.

After some six months of this program, the leakage diminished to maybe a few drops every few days. This was something I could live with. But the best result was that it also broke the depression cycle.

In the meantime, I had learned to rehabilitate my erectile dysfunction with prostaglandin injections. The final aspect of coming to terms with this sort of diagnosis and treatment was to confront and understand the process of grief and loss. We need to know of the four main stages of grief — denial, anger, depression and acceptance. That way, we can learn to accept the new reality of our life.

Adjustment often requires time and re-evaluation of what it means to be a male; it may challenge our belief systems and values, one's faith and the very purpose of being. My aim was to really live a meaningful and contented life. For me, this enlightenment is one of the 'gifts' that a life-threatening condition can reveal.

■ ■ ■ ■

3

'Me too!'
On Loving Someone
With Prostate Cancer

When cancer happens in a family all thoughts go first to the needs and worries of the person who has the cancer. However, in many cases the partners of men with prostate cancer report more distress and worry than do the men themselves. It is hard to know for sure why this is so, and of course all couples will have their own habits of coping and ways of facing challenges. However, it can be the case that watching your partner go through the experience of cancer can seem harder than actually having it.

Standing beside someone you love and watching them undergo painful or difficult procedures and face a threat to their life is heart breaking. You might feel powerless to help. You might not really understand or know what the cancer diagnosis actually means, particularly if you haven't been involved in the doctor's visits or if you haven't discussed this as a couple. If your husband or partner has become withdrawn then you might feel very alone and frustrated in all of this.

Perhaps you feel you are not able to reach out for help — after all you don't have cancer! Many partners have told me that they have felt guilty for wanting support for themselves. You might be the one who takes care of the family's health, and perhaps you tend to put yourself last when it comes to care and attention.

Finally, often in relationships there is one person who is the 'emotional barometer' and who picks up on negative emotion first and takes on the job of easing the tension. If this is you then that is a very big job and it is exhausting!

Partners often report different worries than the patient, and it can be hard to share these when you see your job as being a support person. In my own work, women have told me about worrying how they will manage if their partner dies, especially if they have been married for many years or in a long term relationship. That is a hard fear to share. You might be worried about how you are managing financially now, and what the future might bring, but feel unable to discuss this.

You may have found that in the early phase of the illness you were well supported by friends and family, but that over time you are expected to just 'get on with it'. The experience of prostate cancer is for most a long journey, with ongoing tests and medical checks. So even though treatment might be over, the worry can remain. Coping with treatment side effects can be tough for you too. It might mean that you don't go out as often or see friends as much as you used to. Your sex life will be affected as well and you might be feeling a loss of closeness and physical touch. This might be making you start to feel uncertain about your own attractiveness as a sexual mate.

If the man has experienced a cancer recurrence and is on hormonal blocking medication, there may be stress associated with balancing treatment side effects, quality of life, and controlling the cancer. To say this can be an emotional roller coaster is an understatement.

Looking After Yourself

The first lesson you need to learn and accept is that you matter. Your own wellbeing and mental health remains important for you, as a unique and valuable person in this world. (Yes, this is a lecture just for you!) You also matter for the man who relies on your support, so if you feel you can't look after yourself just for you, then do it for him!

If you are coping well there will be a likely positive flow-on effect to those around you, so make yourself a priority. This might mean scheduling time to do things you find pleasurable, keeping up with your friends, and making time for hobbies and interests.

You also have a right to discuss how you are feeling about the cancer in a private setting with others close to you. This is an important way to seek support that will help you feel less alone and lessen your feelings of distress.

Understanding Coping

In the previous chapter I talked about the importance of understanding your own personal coping style and taking a flexible approach. Do you have a typical approach to problems? How well does this approach usually work for you?

Remember we have already talked a little about the two broad groups of coping approaches: problem solving or emotion focus. Problem solving applies strategies to solve the problem. This is an active approach that gets outcomes and helps you to move forward in a practical and tangible way. An example of problem solving coping as a partner would be to be as informed as you can be about the medical plan. If you are well informed about what the cancer means, what treatments are available, and the likely effects of treatment, then you will feel more confident about being an effective support person. If you are feeling uncertain about what the cancer means you are more likely to worry and feel sad or anxious about the cancer and the future. Being involved in doctor's visits will help. There is also a lot of easy to find information about prostate cancer on the Internet and through phone helplines, so check the appendix in this book for reliable sources of advice.

Emotion focussed coping helps reduce unpleasant emotions. For women this often means talking to their friends or close female family members about what is going on and how they feel. (We rehearse for this as teenagers and young women with endless telephone conversations with our friends!) A good cry helps as well. Emotion focused coping is important and balances and complements problem solving coping.

As described earlier, avoiding thinking (or talking) about the cancer is another type of emotion focussed coping that is often not so helpful, especially for you as a partner and support person. If you avoid a painful issue it gets stronger as a worry — the more you push it away the stronger it will come back. By avoiding a painful problem we can give it more power to hurt us.

Activity

When cancer hits a couple it affects goals in life for both of them. It can seem like a roadblock to long hoped for plans or can make past hopes seem not as important. This can leave you feeling like you have lost control of the ship! Reconnecting with goals and being clear about where you are heading is crucial.

Think about how prostate cancer has affected *your* future goals and hopes. Have your goals changed (or been forgotten) since your partner was diagnosed with cancer? What are the things that matter to you most now in the short-term? Do you have medium- or long-term goals? Perhaps you have lost sight of these in the face of the stress of the cancer and looking after your mate. If so, now is a great time to remember the things that are important to you and, if needed, set new goals.

You might set goals that are about looking after yourself right now. You might have longer term life goals you would like renew and work towards. What would life look like for you in six or twelve months' time in the best of worlds? Write down a list of goals for right now, and for in six months, and for in a year or two. What steps do you need to take to achieve these goals and who can help you with these?

Talk to someone you trust about your most important goals. This will help you confirm your agreement to look after yourself as you deserve. Check your list regularly to see how you are going and revise or change your goals if needed. Again, the main point of this activity is that you have a sense of where you are headed and that you start to place a priority on your own well-being and life happiness without feeling guilty about it.

Now think about how you usually cope with difficulties? What is your main style of coping and how well is this working for you now? Think about a time when you have coped well with a difficult problem and felt pleased with how it turned out. How would you describe your approach then? Now think about a time when you were faced with a problem and it did not go so well. How could you have approached this differently? Are there new coping skills you might need to learn?

Further on in this book you will find more specific advice about ways to look after yourself, and to nurture your relationship with your partner. Feel free to move ahead to chapters that interest you. It will help though if you take the time to reflect about your goals as suggested in this chapter and be clear about where you would like to head.

Personal Stories

Below are personal stories from Avryl and Carole about their experiences when their partners were diagnosed with prostate cancer and the challenges they faced as partners.

Avryl

My husband had a radical prostatectomy in 2009, so it is a few years down the track for me at present, though I still get upset thinking about it even now. I think it was just such a total shock. I was quite young at the time, only 48, and we never saw this coming. I think Graham was very numb when it happened. I played the strong person that I am, but I couldn't help thinking: 'Is he going to die? Am I going to lose him?' It is our second marriage, and we feel we are very lucky that we found each other the second time around. We have a very special bond. Graham is a very special person with a beautiful heart and good values. So when this happened I thought: 'Why him?' It seemed so unfair.

As a woman I think you do want your man to be the strong one to take care of you, and then all of sudden your world is being turned upside down. Definitely, I felt alone and that I couldn't talk to anyone. I didn't think anyone could understand how I was feeling. As well, no one really knew what we were going through because it was all very personal, so we kept a lot of it to ourselves. After his operation, we just thought he would be back to normal so to speak. We didn't get any information to prepare us to deal with his incontinence, or his erectile problems, we had no idea really about what was ahead of us.

After the operation, Graham was incontinent and wearing pads, he felt dirty and not a man anymore, even though I said it didn't worry me. He didn't want to touch me because of how he was feeling, we weren't having sex anymore and I felt unloved and alone. All the romance had gone and we were just living together, almost like we were brother and sister. I was annoying him; maybe we were annoying each other, and we were arguing where we never used to argue, over the stupidest things.

I threw myself into work; it was a way of trying to run away from it all. About twelve months after his surgery I had an anxiety attack at work. I had never had one before and thought I was having a heart attack! It was almost like once he was on the mend I collapsed. I think it was just my body coping with all that was happening. I tend to be like that at times, very strong, on the go, coping with anything that comes along with the biggest of shoulders and then when I stop I just collapse in a heap. I had always felt guilty thinking about me and my needs, because it wasn't about me it was about him. He was the one with the cancer. I'm lucky to have close girlfriends to have some fun with and turn off, but I didn't really talk to them about it. Sometimes I would just burst into tears, and then I would feel like an idiot because I couldn't explain what I was crying about. It was just me letting my emotions go.

Now, I think we have grown as a couple. I think it shows we can face anything. I know our relationship has always been strong but now it's stronger than ever. Though I wouldn't want anyone else to have to go through this.

My main message to partners is to look for support, and feel comfortable to talk and seek help. Going to a support group and getting help from people who know what you are going through makes all the difference. For me, talking to another woman who has been through this was a huge support, and relief. The more you talk about it, the more you see that there are other people in the same situation as you, and you are able to find hope that you will get through it.

Carole

David was diagnosed with prostate cancer in 1999 and it was traumatic for both of us. He was anxious, and his way of dealing with it, at least at first, was to search for alternatives and talk to a lot of people, but not to me. That left me feeling left out and angry. Finally he had his treatment, radical prostatectomy, and then we had his treatment side effects to deal with. It really was a very tough time for him, and for me.

I think I felt lost, totally lost. I remember thinking 'I can't do this'. Looking back I don't think we got very good support from the medical team. I think David kept the physical problems he was struggling with to himself a lot, and we didn't have a good support network around us. It was a second marriage for both of us, so I felt I couldn't talk to the family. I didn't really have anyone I felt I could talk to about it.

I learnt a lot from this experience, about compassion and about caring for others, listening to their stories and then trying to find out where they can get help. I have learnt to look after myself. To help myself relax I put music on to listen to late at night, because I am not the best sleeper, and this helps me wind down. I work, I keep active and listen to the ABC radio every day. It is a distraction from worry and I learn new things about the world all the time.

I think that partners should be involved in the doctors' consultations so everyone is on the same page. I also think we need to have a support service where somebody can talk to couples like David and me, because I think there must lots of people in the exact same situation. As a partner you don't want to take the whole load, you want to share the load. So I guess my advice to couples facing this right now is to talk about it with each other, and if this is hard to do look for someone to help you talk about it. David and I have talked about all this now, and we are great friends, but I wish we had done this earlier. I think it would have made our journey a lot easier.

■■■■

4

'We're in this together'

When cancer happens in a family it affects all of the family in some way. Similarly, when cancer happens to someone who is in a couple relationship, both people in the relationship are affected and how each individual reacts affects the other. This happens on several levels. First, if your partner is very distressed, then that will be distressing to you. By contrast, if your partner is upset but calm, you might find it easier to be calm as well. It is a two-way street, with each person's reaction having some effect on the other. This does not mean that either of you should hide how you feel. In fact, the opposite is true. It is important to be honest and open about how each of you are feeling. The point is to be aware that although you are both individuals with your own unique approach to things, you are connected emotionally.

On another level — and this is the part you can work on together — how each of you copes will affect the other person's experience, and your own. In brief, if people in a couple relationship have a similar approach to coping they tend to have a smoother run.

As an example, if one person wants to talk about the cancer most of the time and the other person prefers to avoid thinking about it until they have to, this can lead to conflict. Similarly, if for the man his main long term goal is to complete treatment and get back to work whereas his partner wants more of a focus on being together and enjoying each others company, both people may feel frustrated and misunderstood.

Something else to consider is that when you are both under pressure (and a prostate cancer diagnosis certainly fits that bill!) it can be harder to get on with each other. You might each feel more sensitive and on the edge, and find that your usual ways of getting over hurdles don't seem to be helping.

It is not that one person is right and the other wrong, just that their individual approaches to the situation are different. It is this difference that can make the journey harder.

So, if no one is right or wrong what can you do? The key is effective communication. By that I mean communication that allows each person to have a say and feel heard and with both partners working together as a team. What is also important is remembering that you are both under a lot of stress dealing with the cancer, so things that might in the past have been easy to solve can seem tougher. In this situation, putting more effort into how you communicate with each other can make all the difference.

Communicating Effectively With Your Partner

Perhaps the first thing to try and avoid is mind reading. This goes both ways. In relationships we often act as if we can read our partners' minds and they can read ours. We think we know why our partner is angry or upset, even though we haven't checked it out with them, and more often than not we think it is all about us. Or we think that our partner should know how we want to be supported and that if they don't give us what we need then they don't really care or aren't interested.

Compounding the problem, we mind read and then treat our conclusions as if they are fact, and react accordingly, even if the trigger issue is actually quite trivial. Who has never thought of their partner: 'If he/she really loved me they would have done the dishes/put out the rubbish/picked up the dry cleaning?'

The first step then is to accept that although you may know your partner better than anyone else in the world, you have never known them under quite these circumstances and that unless you have clairvoyant skills you cannot read their mind. The only way you can know for sure what they are thinking or worrying about is if they let you know. Until you check out your assumptions they are just your fantasies, not fact.

In reverse then, unless your partner has clairvoyant skills they also cannot read your mind, and expecting them to do so will most likely not get you what you want or need.

So my tip is that first, you need to decide as a couple if you want to work on improving how you communicate. If the answer is 'yes' then you need to agree to work at this together in a non-judgmental and supportive way. By this I mean accepting that you are both unique individuals and that each of you has the right to feel the way you do and that these feelings are not right or wrong, they just are what they are. It is useful to remember here that men and women often have quite different ways of coping with problems: men may tend to want to act and fix things and women are more likely to want to talk about the issue. In prostate cancer support groups when I have talked about this I have suggested that men are giraffes and women are zebras! Both are beautiful creatures but in the plains they act quite differently — although they will both run from a big scary predator!

If you both accept that being different is okay then the next step is to try sharing some of those feelings and talking to each other about what they mean for you. For each of you this might mean first up sharing what your main worry is and how you feel you are coping. Talking this over and then checking with each other to make sure you are both clear about the other person's perspective is central to good communication. You might share how you have been feeling over the past two to three weeks, what thoughts have been worrying you the most, and what seems to help you feel calmer or less stressed.

Once you are clear about where you each are at in terms of your main worries, a good next step might be to check if there are things you can do to help each other cope. Clear and practical suggestions are best (for example, 'if I am upset just hug me and don't try and solve anything' is better than 'just be there for me' or 'if I need to go out to the shed for a while to be on my own, let me have some space but then come down in an hour or so with a cup of tea' is better than 'stop fussing').

What if talking makes it worse?

Sometimes cancer can feel overwhelming for a couple. This is more likely if the relationship is still new and perhaps not so solid yet, or if you have had troubles in the past. As well, if you have other pressing problems to cope with at the same time, such as money worries or children or aging parents who need a lot of support from you, the pressure can seem huge.

Getting to the bottom of things without blaming each other for the situation you are in can be hard. You might need to think back to the things that brought you together in the first place, what it is about each other that you most value, and what are the things now as a couple that bind you together. Are these things still present for you? Are they important? If the answer is 'yes' then reminding yourselves of your shared core values can help you get back a sense of being a team.

Next, remember, the experience of a cancer diagnosis is a major life stress. It doesn't get much tougher than this. So give each other a break and try not to be hard on yourself and your partner. Try and work flexibly on problems and to see each other's points of view. Treat yourself and your partner with kindness.

Finally, if you feel you cannot get on top of this as a couple, seek help. Talking to an experienced, couples focussed psychologist or counsellor can make all the difference.

Activity

Set aside time (about 20 minutes) once or twice each week to talk with each other about how you each are feeling and coping — no problem solving, just listening and making sure you have checked you understand and 'get it'.

The rules are don't judge or criticise and don't interrupt.

Next, think of three to five things your partner could do to support you. Make a commitment to each other to try these out and see how it goes. Be clear about which support action matters the most to each of you.

Be fair.

Finally, take time to do a pleasurable activity with each other that has nothing to do with cancer. By making each other a priority you will strengthen your feelings of connectedness and you might even have some fun!

Personal Stories

Below are personal stories from two different couples. Jan and Gordon talk about how weekly meetings helped them keep in touch with what was going on for each other. Jim and Laura found that being patient and accepting each other as they are was crucial. For both couples, taking time to communicate about what was going on became central to their approach in managing the challenges of cancer as a team.

Gordon

I was diagnosed with prostate cancer in early 2004. My PSA was elevated —it was 20 — and after a course of antibiotics it was still going up. The next step was a biopsy that came back positive. Because my PSA was high, radiation therapy seemed a better option that surgery, and so I ended up having high dose brachytherapy, external beam radiation therapy, with a course of hormone treatment that went on for two years after treatment. My PSA stayed down for a couple of years and then started to rise again. As a result I am now back on hormone treatment and participating in a clinical trial for a new set of drugs. Jan says I rattle with all the pills I am on!

It was pretty rough finding out about the cancer. We came to the point of just accepting I've got cancer and it's not going to go away. We went through a period of having weekly meetings when we would sit down on Saturday mornings and write down what we were going to do, and what were our worries, and things like that. We did this for quite a while.

It is important to work out ways of communicating, because, particularly with men, we are blokes and we don't want to talk about it! But it is necessary to talk about things. Sometimes it is easier to talk to people who are not your spouse or partner. I had a couple of friends that were in the same situation and we had conversations that I wouldn't have been able to have with Jan at the time. But since then we have been able to work it so that now the conversations that Jan and I have are the same sort of conversations I had with my friends. I think with me it was getting the confidence to actually say what was on my mind. Partnerships are made by two people trying to work through a system of what happens and losing a fear that if you say how you feel you might appear to be less a person in your partner's eyes. It is important to be able to actually say this is how I feel or this is the way it is for me at the moment, and have enough trust that it will be seen and supported.

I think part of it is you are brought up to say as boys, particularly of our vintage, that you are the male and you have to be seen as strong and out there.

Jan

When Gordon and I were doing our weekly meetings we would tell our friends. They thought we were mad, but it was really important. We were bogged down, we were a ship without a rudder and didn't know what to do and where to go. Gordon was really lost saying: 'What do I do? What don't I do?' Making time for good quality honest conversation, even if your list starts off with 'when is the fence going to get repaired?' or 'when is the pool man coming?' or whatever it is, gives you a structure to deal with the 'don't know' stuff that sometimes you don't deal with because it's all too hard.

We do have rows — differences of opinion — but for us that's about honest discussion and not avoiding the difficult stuff. I don't sit down with Gordon and say, 'Right, we are going to have an honest discussion now'. It's about when the time is right, you sit and say 'listen there is something we need to have a conversation about'. For me it's trying to gauge when it's the right time to have that discussion and how far the conversation can go. I think at the end of the day Gordon appreciates the fact that we do put the hard stuff on the table and this gives him a chance to talk about where he is coming from and how it feels, 'cause he is a bloke and they tend not to talk about feelings and hopes and goals and aspirations.

Jim

I was diagnosed with prostate cancer in 2007 and was put straight away on hormone therapy, external beam radiation and then high dose brachytherapy. I was on the hormone treatment for over 6 months all told, and that was the worst. I suppose most blokes would say the lack of sex drive was a big concern, but I found it was the all the other effects. You start to lose muscle, you don't feel too enthusiastic, you're moody, you end up having some memory loss.

I stopped work immediately and we had 5 acres at the time and then not long after I decided that we would sell it because Laura wouldn't be able to deal with it. I was getting the property ready for sale so that occupied my mind a fair bit and gave me something else to think about, but it was pretty tough times. I remember, and I often talk about this, Laura was still teaching and she came home one day and I was sitting out the back on a park bench that we had and she came round the corner of the house and I was sitting there crying my eyes out and she said 'What's wrong with you?' I said 'I need a dog. I am sitting here by myself, no one to talk to, you are off at work, and I am feeling miserable.' So we ended up going and finding a dog, which gave me something else to distract myself. When we got that little pup that was the best move we made. That was probably the worst I got, just that short period.

Laura didn't say anything at the time, but later on told me that while I was on the hormone treatment I didn't have any affection for her. I didn't really notice that I wasn't paying her any attention. Because of the effects of the drug, it was normal for me, I wasn't interested in sex or having a relationship or cuddling her or anything like that. All interest in Laura was gone; we were just two people walking around the same house. She felt really unloved.

Things didn't turn around until I went off the hormone treatment and we slowly got back to normal. It just took time. Then in 2008 we did a personal development course together to help us in some volunteering work we were doing. It really came out then, to talk about things not just think about them, and we found our relationship improved so much. It helped us to understand each other better, each of us do certain things, and that we each have positives and negatives. So you just work to focus on the positives and reduce the negatives, and being aware of yourself, what you are thinking and how you are acting.

In this situation you need to talk to each other, that is the main thing, involve your wife, from diagnosis onwards. Every time I go to the doctors Laura goes with me, goes in to the consultation, and gets all the information as well. If I have to go for scans or anything, Laura goes with me and she's there and supports me 100% all the way and she was like that from the very beginning.

You need to be patient about sex. Gradually over time after I came off the hormone therapy it came back. I wasn't on the hormone therapy for too long, the longer you are on it, the longer it takes to get back and you have to be really patient. There are other ways to be affectionate though and you need to look at all that and be aware that you have a partner and they have needs too. And don't blame yourself; it's not your fault.

Laura

As a partner, I am not going through what Jim is going through personally and I don't know exactly what he is going through. I mean, I can see it, but I can't actually feel it. Jim's pretty positive and because of that I think it does help him a lot. I suppose I try to be happy and try to do things and have a variety of things that we do together — go places not just mope around the house.

I didn't get any support when Jim was diagnosed. We didn't really know what we were doing and we panicked! Now with what we know I think both of us would have stayed still for a bit, held back and tried to come to terms with it more.

I do think that in a partnership you both need to be really involved. We did notice that a lot of men at medical consultations were there on their own. We would go to the doctors and see men sitting in the waiting room on their own, or sometimes if the wives did come, they would just sit out in the waiting room while the husband went in to see the doctor. I think partners should find out as much as they can about what is going on, because if you don't ask the questions, sometimes the doctor is not going to tell you.

■ ■ ■ ■

5

How to Make Decisions You can Live With

Imagine you own a sleek red Ferrari. You have owned and loved it for years, driven it a bit too hard and fast at times, neglected it a little of late, and you recently noticed a vague knock in the engine. You take it to a specialist mechanic, a little embarrassed about the state of the duco, but determined to get it fixed and back on the road. The mechanic runs a few tests and says it is actually a pretty serious mechanical problem and he offers you four different options. First, he suggests you could just let it go for a while and see what happens. It might not cause you too much trouble, you could wait and see. Or if you really want to just get if fixed he has three different approaches that he thinks will all do the job. Each of these three approaches has different possible issues in terms of how long the car will be off the road, the cost, how long the engine will likely go trouble free, and what might need to be done if the problem recurs. The mechanic gives you a leaflet with all the options and sends you home to think about it.

Sound familiar? It can be a big shock when you are diagnosed with prostate cancer and find out that there are several different treatment options and that you need to be involved in the decision about what treatment to have. This might sound crazy at first. If your car is broken the mechanic usually tells you what needs to be done. That is their job after all. Similarly, you might expect one correct 'fix' to treat a cancer and you probably expect the doctor to offer you this one best way. Being asked to make this decision yourself is a big call.

One of the first challenges is the medical language that doctors use. Maybe you didn't even really know you had a prostate gland before this, much less exactly where it is (so close to the plumbing) and what it does. The words used to describe cancer and treatments are unfamiliar to most people. Who (other than health professionals) uses words like *carcinoma, radical prostatectomy*, and *brachytherapy* in normal day-to-day life? It can be hard to be sure about exactly what the doctor is telling you and what it really means. As well, much of what you will be told is expressed in numbers, percentages or chances of things happening. Even doctors don't always understand these risk estimates, so how hard is it then for a lay person?

Statistics can be misleading and confusing. For example, if you are told that having an extra type of treatment will reduce your chance of the cancer coming back by 50% that sounds pretty worthwhile. But if your chance of the cancer coming back is only 8%, then what the extra drug does is cut that by half to 4%. You might still think this is a path worth taking, but you can see how 50% sounds so much better than 4%. If you read that after surgery the chance of not being able to get an erection is 30%, does that mean you might not get an erection 30% of the time or does it mean three out of ten men won't be able to get an erection? How do you know your chances of being in the 30% anyway?

Aside from being confusing to many, the other thing about percentages and risk numbers, is that while they will be the best figures available, they are based on trials and large groups of other people. Not you. So they are an estimate of what might happen, not what will happen. So the uncertainty remains.

Making Decisions under Stress

As a rule we don't think as clearly when we are stressed, and you don't get much more stress than when you are facing cancer. If you think back to the analogy of a diagnosis of prostate cancer as 'facing a tiger', you are getting ready from a physiological point of view to fight or run. This stress response, as it is often called, is designed to help you keep yourself safe from immediate danger. It is not designed to help you sit down and reflect clearly on all possible actions you might take, weigh up and consider the pros and cons of different approaches, and then choose a carefully laid out plan. Our thinking just does not work as well when we are stressed. If you think of your mind as your work bench, when you are stressed your 'mental work bench' becomes cluttered. It becomes harder to find things, to make sense of them, and to make a decision. This means that while for many men and their partners they would prefer a quickly achieved clear plan of action so they can move out of uncertainty and get on with it, this is often not possible.

Ways to Make Decisions

Most of us do not have brains that work like computers — in a programmed, predictive, and logical way. We are much more complicated and interesting than that. The way we make decisions is influenced by our feelings, attitudes, past history, what has worked well for us in the past, and how important the decision is.

There are two approaches people tend apply when making decisions. There is the *systematic* approach, and then there is the *quick short cut.*

In the systematic approach we carefully gather information, look at the pros and cons, weigh it all up, and then make a call. Systematic decision making takes effort and time. It can mean a better informed decision where you are very clear about the choice you made and why. This is the type of decision making approach often seen as best. An approach where you are well informed about your options, involved in the decision in an equal partnership with your doctor and with the support of the people most close to you. On the other hand, if you have an information overload it can be easy to get lost and to focus on issues that seem important but actually aren't. As well, taken to the extreme there is a point where the searching for information can become a type of avoidance — avoiding a decision by looking for certainty or an answer that just isn't there.

If we choose to go for the quick short cut instead we usually look for a cue that we might choose to follow. An example would be going for the same option as someone you admire or respect, or who got a good result from their choice. Short cut decision making strategies are very useful to have as they are quick and require less effort than the systematic approach. A possible pitfall though is if you use a short cut and it doesn't work out well, you might later wish you have taken a different approach.

Some people tend to be more systematic, others go more for cues, most of us do a bit of both. How important the decision is and how confident you feel about your ability to make the decision will also influence how you approach the decision.

As an example, when you bought your last car, did you read up on all the latest car reviews, compile a list all the features that mattered most to you and then match these to each possible car choice? Did you then run a series of test drives and then finally make a choice based on weighing up the pros and cons of each car? If you did, then that was an example of systematic decision making. Or, did you buy a Holden because you are a Holden man and always have been or choose a Toyota because most of your friends drive one and they think they are the most reliable? Both of these last two examples are short cuts.

So how should I make my decision?

In the best of worlds you would start by being well informed about your cancer, clear about how much support you need in making the decision from your doctor and your family, and then you would use your support people to help you work this through. A few tips are:

- Take your time. There is seldom a need to make an immediate decision. Talk to your doctor and be clear about your best timeline.
- Be informed. Read up about prostate cancer from reliable sources such as those listed in the Appendix of this book.
- Talk about the decision with your specialist and maybe your GP, and if you are still unclear go back and ask more questions.
- Feel very comfortable about getting a second opinion if you feel you want an alternative view. You have a right to a second opinion and most doctors are happy to organise this for you.
- It can be helpful to tape your discussions with your

doctor to listen to again at home in case you missed important details.

- Take a support person with you to your doctor's visits, two heads are better than one!
- Contact a support group and talk to men who have had different treatments so you can get the personal view.
- Be wary of uninformed opinions that can throw you off track

Activity

Make a list of the treatments your doctor has suggested would be suitable for you. Beside each option list the possible positives (the pros) and the possible negatives (the cons).

Looking at the pros and cons for each, does it look like one option has more pros and fewer cons than the others?

Now put a circle around the pros that matter to you most and the cons that worry you the most. What option looks like it will get you what you value most?

Take this list to your doctor and talk it over with him to make sure you have the facts right. Talk the list over with your partner or someone close to you that you trust. This will help you clarify further what option seems to be closest to your values and will keep your support network in the loop.

Will I regret my decision?

Without a crystal ball it is not possible to know for sure how you will feel about your decision down the track. However, if you take time and make a carefully considered choice you will know, whatever happens, that you made the best choice you could in a tough situation.

Personal Stories

Below are personal stories from Geoff and Allan about how they each approached making their decisions about treatment, and how they feel about that decision now.

Geoff

I was diagnosed in 2009, and had a radical prostatectomy and dissection of my lymph glands. It was an anxious time, with uncertainty about what the cancer meant for me, and I was also worried about the idea of having surgery. I have had previous problems with deep vein thrombosis, so I was a high risk for surgery in terms of possible complications. So it was a real issue to work out what would be the best treatment for me and how this would affect my partner Barbara. We were both involved in all the consultations, the decision making and all the follow-up. Prayer was very important for both myself and my wife at this time as well.

I read a lot of medical articles, but these articles can't tell you about you as an individual. They are studies about groups of men. What we needed was discussions with the specialists about what the studies meant for us. We saw a total of three doctors — two urologists, they were very different, and I also saw a radiation oncologist. With the second urologist we came away feeling very comfortable with the decision which we discussed at the time and really felt as comfortable as one can with the prospect of surgery. We felt that we had been able to talk and ask questions and the questions were answered, and discussed in a very easy way. It made so much difference for both of us, it really did.

I was well informed and as I said, read up a lot, first about the surgery and the risks involved and how to minimise those. We did a fair bit of work on that and then about the possible side effects of the surgery. It is difficult to get a balance. I think blokes are in two groups, one are men who want surgery and want it removed and external to them. Then the other are men who won't have a bar of surgery and go for the other options. I was worried about incontinence and erectile dysfunction but it is difficult to actually get a balanced view of all the pros and cons. You know that there are some risks but percentages aren't always easy to understand or helpful. What you can do is find out what the risks are as precisely as you can, through reading and talking to the surgeon, and from this getting a ball park figure of what you might be facing.

In the end for me the big issues were surviving surgery without complications and then facing erectile dysfunction and urinary incontinence. I was at first keen on brachytherapy from the sex point of view, but I thought it would be big trouble because of the urinary difficulty I was having at the time. I chose surgery because I felt surgery would be the only definitive way of knowing the extent of my cancer, and secondly I was already having urinary problems, difficulty passing water, and I thought that the prostatectomy would get rid of that. I still think this was the best decision for me.

My advice to others is work on this together, take your time and seek more than one opinion. Be sure you are comfortable with what is happening. Talk to as many people as can, and if you have a support group in your area give it a try. There will be people there who have been through that journey and really have heaps of knowledge and can answer a lot of your questions. Be comfortable with your doctor, and if you are in a relationship make sure you both know what is going on. This is something that affects you both and it is really important that you are both in the decision making.

Allan

At the time I was diagnosed with prostate cancer my awareness of the disease was based on the experience of a close friend from my engineering student days. While our lives had taken different paths we were still in contact and I did learn from John in his late 50s that he had undergone a radical prostatectomy and he was getting on with life. 'The disease is easy to diagnose' he advised, 'and you can do something about it if diagnosed with it'

Just prior to my diagnosis, city based GP medical centres were starting up and based entirely on the improved flexibility and convenience of securing an appointment I had decided not to remain with the GP who bought out my retiring GP's practice. The very next time I needed the services of a GP I went to the clinic closest to my office. That occurred on a Saturday morning when consultations were provided without appointment by one of the two doctors rostered on. I was feeling feverish and quite unwell.

I was attended to by a mid-30s female GP. As one component of the consultation, and because I had arrived without any of my medical history, I was asked to undergo a series of tests at a nearby private hospital. One definitive piece of information relevant to this story identified that my PSA was high for my age. While that condition was in no way connected to the medical situation that I was experiencing at the time it did lead on to a visit to a urologist, a DRE and a biopsy. Even though I was entirely without any physical or other symptoms associated with having prostate cancer its existence was definitively confirmed.

Before my first appointment with the urologist I heard a community announcement over the radio that a prostate cancer support group was to be held that night. I went along. It was the first of many steps on the journey that I took to become as informed as possible about prostate cancer, treatment options, implications of side effects of treatment, treatment impacts on my employment, emotional highs and lows, survivor stories and survival statistics.

When my prostate cancer was confirmed I was already conditioned to accept that possibility purely on the statistical possibility when considered within the context of my sex and age range. I was 65 years of age. Gaining an understanding that the cancer's characteristics did have a logical structure was an engaging experience. Most of its descriptors are defined either numerically, or in relative terms — the PSA, the Gleason Score, the Stage of the disease, the volume of the prostate, the number of biopsy cores that were positive, and the urine flow. That awareness was comforting because we engineers work well with stats and I found that my predicament could be somewhat demystified!

Treatment options in my community were relatively limited at that time — essentially open surgery, radiation or hormone therapy. I was advised by the urologist that for my particular circumstances I would be a good candidate for either surgery or radiation. My overall health and fitness were good and there were no physical or emotional situations that might have complicated the choice of treatment. The prediction was that I could expect very similar outcomes from either of the two available treatments of surgery and external beam radiation therapy. Through the above interaction with the urologist I gained a reasonable understanding of how the surgery option would impact on my daily living, my post treatment recovery and my return to work.

At that time I was working on an assignment that required intermittent on-site involvement in a regional country area. I obtained a comparable consultation from a radiation oncologist and formed the view that the radiation option offered scope for lifestyle considerations appropriate to my circumstances that the surgery option precluded. Radiation did not require me to cease working for any treatment at any time. If I took this option I could continue my pattern of early gym workouts three mornings a week. I could also vary the timing of treatment sessions to suit my schedule

Accordingly, the decision to choose radiation for my treatment was made on lifestyle factors that were important to my family and me at the time. To me, prostate cancer was not immediately life threatening. The impact was decidedly more life confronting. Just what was I being required to deal with? Where would I get the information and support that I would require? Who were the specialists that I would consult with — the professionals, and those with lived experiences?

I was being required to make a call on what I understood, not the whole spectrum of what was involved. In life, engineers can be required to make important decisions on a daily basis. They work within the context of a whole range of competencies provided by others on whom we routinely rely — designers, manufacturers and operators. So what is so different in terms of process about deciding on your choice of treatment for your prostate cancer?

I took three months to decide on my choice of treatment. I took advice from health care professionals, I listened to the experiences of men who had travelled the journey before me, and I took account of life style choices that were important to me and my family. No medical practitioner could have made that decision for me. I did not deliberate at length on possible side effects of treatment that might be experienced down the track. I felt the downsides of worrying about what you just don't know could have a greater negative impact on me than the disease itself.

I made the decision that determined the start of my prostate cancer journey of treatment and survival success. At the same time I made a commitment to prepare myself to deal with issues not yet defined, as and when it became important for me to do so, and that would involve ongoing inclusion of health care specialists, desk research and learning from others who were still travelling a journey that I had yet to experience.

■■■■

6

Sex: 'What now?'

Sex is important. Without reproduction we would eventually cease to exist. The survival of the human race depends on sex. This means that biologically as adults we are all at some level sexual beings, even if we are not in a sexual relationship. As thinking beings though (with large brains) there is for all of us a more complicated social side to sex.

We are bombarded much of the time with messages about sex. If we go to the movies or watch television there is a good chance we will see a warning about nudity and sexual references, which most of us don't even always notice. We have advertisements on bill-boards and television and in magazines from people trying to sell us things by inferring that there is a link between sex and their product. The messages include: 'If we wear this deodorant, drive this car or motorbike, or even if we live in a certain type of apartment, then we will be sexier and more successful in love. While we kind of know these ads aren't really true, who has never succumbed wishfully and given it a go?

These days its pretty hard to get away from sex, or the idea of sex, no matter what our background or views are around this sensitive topic. Sex is ubiquitous.

However, despite all this exposure (and how important sex is for the species) for many of us sex is not an easy topic to talk about. This is somewhat ironic given how much time in our lives we spend thinking about it, avoiding it, worrying about it, looking for it, or enjoying it! As we grow up we learn a lot of rules about sex (often unspoken but clear nonetheless) from our parents and our peers. This includes rules about what sort of sex is okay, when it is okay and with whom, and how we should think or talk about sex. These rules have a big influence on how we manage sex in our lives, and they are not always helpful to us. This may be even more so when sex and making love becomes difficult or more complicated because of cancer treatments or because our bodies are aging and have started to work a little differently. When this happens we need to learn new ways of having sex, but communicating and experimenting often do not come naturally.

How Sex Might Change

Let's start with aging. It is a fact that as we age our sexual responses change.

For women, decreases in the female sex hormones as they go through menopause can make sex less pleasurable. Vaginal lubrication often decreases and the lining of the vagina thins and is less elastic, making penetration tight or painful.

Sexual desire or libido may also decrease, although life stress may be more important than hormones in women's interest and energy for sex. If you are not in the mood or sex is painful, it can be harder to reach an orgasm.

As well as this, let's be honest, we live in a culture that celebrates youth as beauty and idealizes younger women. In these times as an older woman you can feel a bit invisible. As we age our whole body changes in other ways, and it's not just our hormones. Gravity hits, fat starts to appear in unhelpful places, and we start to lose muscle tone and strength. It is hard to feel interested in sex and romance if you feel sexually unattractive or uninteresting and not valued in this way.

Men experience changes as well. Although men get more leeway to look 'distinguished' as they age, gravity hits everyone, and men also may get more fat around the middle, and lose some muscle — the usual list for all but the super fit. Testosterone also declines with age, especially in men who are not physically fit. Sexual desire is often not as strong and the amount of ejaculate is less. It can take longer to get an erection and your erection may not be as strong or as persistent and orgasms can at times seem less intense. In men, the ability to get and keep hard erections is closely tied to cardiovascular (blood vessel) health. Men who have high blood pressure, diabetes, clogged arteries, a lot of belly fat, and who smoke or drink too much alcohol are much more likely to get erection problems with aging.

All of this is going on for men and women at just the age when prostate cancer is most likely to hit. And then we discover that perhaps the most pronounced negative physical effect of prostate cancer treatments is on sex.

How Prostate Cancer affects Sex

The prostate gland sits snugly around the base of the bladder and so is right in the middle of the nerves and blood supply needed for an erection. This means that surgery and radiation therapy for prostate cancer can have a direct effect on a man's ability to get or maintain an erection. There are plenty of easy to find booklets and web pages that outline exactly how and why this happens, but this is the nub of it. A man might find after treatment that he is unable to get or keep a hard erection, or that his erections are unreliable. This can be devastating. If a man has radiation therapy for a time orgasms might be painful and for all men who have had treatment, the amount of ejaculate will lessen or after surgery to remove the prostate be completely dry.

If a man is on hormone blocking treatment, he will find his desire for sex reduces as well as his erections, making it even more difficult to keep an active, pleasurable sex life.

It is important to be clear about this: these are physical treatment effects. They are not 'in your head' and to solve them, you will probably need to use medical treatments. There are a range of pills, medicines that can be injected into the penis, sexual aids like vacuum pumps, and even surgery to put a penile implant (pump system) inside a man's body. The main point is that this is something that will require medical help. As well, many doctors now advise that getting the blood flow back to the penis early in recovery is important for long term erectile function. So thinking about this sooner rather than later is a good idea.

There is a psychological side as well though. The worry of a cancer diagnosis itself can reduce sexual interest, just as you might have found when other tough things have happened in your life. Many men report feeling that if they can't get an erection they are not sexually interesting or capable and that this stops them from even thinking sexy thoughts.

Finally, sex after prostate cancer needs more planning, understanding, and communication within a couple, as well as medical help. If lovemaking doesn't work so well in the early days some couples find they feel less inclined to persist in trying and they just give up.

Why bother?

This is really up to you. Some couples do say that they had become less interested in sex before the cancer anyway and that they have talked it over now and decided it was time to give away having sex. For these couples, physical closeness, affection and comfort stays an important part of their lives with cuddling, kissing and lots of hugs becoming their main way of keeping physically close and connected.

For other couples, keeping an active sex life matters. If you want to stay sexually active, or you can see that your partner is frustrated about sex, there is lots you can do. The key things are to talk about it, be informed, be patient with each other, flexible in your approach and open to new things — and to start early. The sooner you get to work on this the more likely you will be to succeed.

How do we get started?

When all this is going on it is easy for a couple to have misunderstandings about sex. A man who is worried about whether he can perform sexually might become withdrawn and stop initiating sex. His partner however might see this as rejection and feel hurt and frustrated. Talking honestly with each other about how sex and love making has changed for you both, and how you would each like sex to be is the first step.

The next step is to be informed about the physical effects of prostate cancer treatments and what treatments and aids are available to help you with these effects. Some useful resources are listed in the Appendix in this book. Your doctor will have advice and be able to guide you about what treatments might work best for you and may also refer you to a doctor who specialises in sexual health.

Sex is a mutual activity, so if you are in a relationship you need to work on this as a couple. This means at the outset talking with each other about the options you have and working out which might suit you both best. In the previous chapter I talked about ways to make informed decisions about treatment, and these strategies can be applied here as well. In brief, this means be clear about and list your options, work out the pros and con, weigh up what you think suits you both best, work closely with your doctor on the plan, and be ready to change the plan as needed. Too many men try a treatment for a sexual problem but give up when it does not restore them right away to their memories of being age twenty. You and your partner may need to try several different treatments before you find one that satisfies you both.

This does not mean though that you should turn having sex into work. When you do put the plan in place make sure to also do the fun romantic things to add a little zing. It does not have to mean a second honeymoon. Just putting a high priority on time for talking, maybe a nice dinner, dancing in the dark to romantic music, or watching a sexy movie, and above all plenty of time and privacy.

Be aware that being anxious about having sex after prostate cancer is normal, but may not be helpful. Taking time to keep physical closeness a part of your life without feeling pressured about sexual performance is crucial. Remember that sex does not have to include penetration. Many couples find other ways to give each other sexual pleasure that is both satisfying and helps them keep a feeling of being physically close and intimate. This is what this chapter's Activity is about.

Activity

Set aside time to talk about how you are each feeling about your sexual lives and how you would like things to be in the best of worlds. This is best not done in the bedroom, where you might each feel a little tense. Try talking about this over a cup of coffee or a relaxing drink after dinner. You need privacy and to pick a time when you won't be interrupted. The goal here is to agree on what steps you would like to take as a couple to get sex back on track. Once you agree, you can start to make a plan about what external medical help you would like, get informed about the options, and try out options that suit you both. Think of your options as a menu (perhaps French!) to choose from. Be prepared to try different approaches until you find one that you are both happy with.

When you are trying to get back to a normal sex life, it helps to start by making time to give each other physical sensual pleasure without having actual sex. For this activity sexual touch is banned! Set aside at least one hour for private physical touch time. You need a private place like your bedroom, there needs to be no interruptions, and you both need to agree that the next hour (or two) is for giving and receiving pleasure through physical touch. Candles, soft mood lighting and relaxing music is a good start as well as a state of undress to the extent you are comfortable. Now take turns touching and massaging your partner in non-sexual places, fifteen to twenty minute turns each. Notice how good it feels to touch and be touched, and to give and receive pleasure. Talk to each other (compliments are good) and have fun with this. This exercise is about being close and feeling good about yourself and each other.

When you are comfortable with touching in places that are less 'sexual', try different ways of giving and receiving sexual pleasure short of having actual sexual intercourse. This can include touching each other on the breasts and 'private parts' and giving pleasure through physical stimulation using hands or your mouth. Be playful. Instead of worrying about reaching an orgasm, just focus on learning new ways to give each other pleasure. Ask each other what feels good and work on learning what kinds of touch your partner prefers. For this exercise sexual intercourse is not the goal. The goal is finding ways to give sexual pleasure to each other that do not rely on having an erection or achieving penetration.

Personal Stories

Below are personal stories from Barbara and Geoff about how they approached getting their sexual life back on track after treatment; and a story with a touch of humour in it from Ian whose main message is get on to it early!

Barbara

Geoff had a radical prostatectomy in 2009, and my feelings at the time focussed on getting rid of the cancer. My concerns were for Geoff at the actual time of the surgery and for his health during the operation, but also what was going to happen afterwards, and how were we going to cope.

Our sex life was great; it was really exciting and really good. The idea of how that was going to work after surgery I suppose wasn't initially worrying me, but afterwards was more on my mind. We didn't address this until well after surgery, we just thought we could do something about it if we found Geoff couldn't get an erection afterwards. I heard a lot about the various things you can do, but we didn't go into the detail. It didn't seem relevant, and we thought we would we just have to tackle that when we came to it.

We were able to get a lot of comprehensive information about couple and sexuality issues from a couples support trial we were in, and that helped us through enormously. We worked through the information independently and then talked about it as a couple. The way it was presented and authored was terrific. We also had the opportunity to speak together for perhaps an hour at a time and share the issues that were concerning us with a mentor that was so important. I think it made a lot of difference to our openness with one another.

The mentor also gave us practical tips, like talking more, taking out time for us as a couple. Our lives were busy and still are busy. But making a special time in our week, in our day, to talk about our sex life, things we can try, how did it work for each one of us, what was good, what was not so good, this really helped. Listening more to one another as well, that also made a huge difference. These are very practical ideas, things that we thought we were doing pretty well to be honest. But having a mentor and having someone else to share with made us realise that there was more we could do.

Support groups can help as well, I know in our own support group people are very open in talking about sexual issues and the problems that they are facing.

I think openness and genuineness, being genuine with each other is really, really important. You can't afford to hold back. I think you have to be quite open about sex and I can understand how people could find that very difficult. For me, this is essential as part of being a couple, having a partner, and having someone to share your life with.

Geoff

We have always been very open in talking about sex, and everything else as far as that goes. When we went back to the surgeon for the six week check-up we started to ask what we could be doing to help matters along. Indeed at that stage we saw a colleague of my urologist who took us for an hour to talk about what we might be able to do.

I think as a first step you have to talk about it with each other. You've got to be prepared; I mean it can't come as a great shock or surprise. You have to think through about what you want as a couple before you embark and discuss it with the doctor.

One practical thing that I think is very relevant is to see a specialist about it. We saw a surgeon who suggested I see a colleague of his who specialised in erectile problems. We spent a long time with that fellow talking about what we could do about it, right from the start, right after the post operative visit. It was very helpful.

I agree with Barbara that the support trial reinforced everything that we thought we had been doing, but refocused us at a time when we had tried some things about erectile dysfunction and things hadn't been going too well. It brought us back to address the issue and actually made us make some progress. The mentor also gave us some very practical tips which helped us to make progress on the matter. We could have dropped it at that stage and said 'oh well, you know that's it for sex'. But we persevered through that and got some support to give us the means and strategies to solve the sexual problems we faced. Rather that thinking we've hit a dead end, we thought there were some other avenues to explore. We also got some very good tips from the counsellor about the penile injections and the vacuum pump.

It was really worth the effort and focus and now we are very happy with how things are going in this area our lives. But we do have to stay focussed and we don't take it for granted.

Ian

I underwent a robotic prostatectomy in May 2009. I went through the usual urinary leakage (more like a flood at times) which gradually decreased. After six months I began to feel like having sex again, however I could not get much of an erection and certainly could not maintain it for long when I did manage to have a partial one. I tried Viagra and other pills, and a vacuum pump which didn't help. I looked at penile injections but decided I didn't want to go sticking those in my penis (it had had enough I thought).

As time went on with no improvement I became very angry and morose. I had been through all this just to face impotency. My relationship with my wife deteriorated and my work suffered. Approximately nine months after the operation, I went to see my urologist for a check up and asked him about an implanted pump. His reaction was that there was no need. All I really needed were the injections and that they weren't the issue I had built them up to be. He gave me a referral to a men's health doctor. I think I made the appointment as I was walking out his door.

My first encounter with this men's health doctor was a revelation and a riot. He spent some time explaining the process in detail and then he showed me how to inject myself. We started with a dosage just under the maximum. There it was — a thing of beauty and a joy forever (well the forever part was right). After I had gloried in the sensation for some time he convinced me that I should inject the antidote. I then left his office (both hands in my pockets) and went back to my own office. The doctor had given me tablets to take if the erection did not go away. It didn't, so I took the tablets and then remembered that I had a meeting scheduled with two women. It was too late to cancel!

With a strategically placed manila folder I entered the meeting room, quickly sat down and made sure that my errant and rampant erection was securely out of sight under the table. At the end of the meeting (still rampant) I then had to juggle shaking hands, saying goodbye and the manila folder. I then made a beeline to my office and phoned the doctor. I returned to his office (both hands in my pockets) and he gave me another injection of antidote.

After that I experimented with lower and lower dosage levels until I had worked out what was the best for a comfortable erection that went away after a reasonable time. My sex life and my attitude improved exponentially. Over three years from the original operation I still use small doses of the serum for a fantastic result. If I had had the courage to bring the subject up directly with my urologist and started the injections earlier I would not have gone through so much mental turmoil and my life would have returned to normal much more quickly. My advice, don't put it off!

■■■■

'I think therefore I am!' (cogito ergo sum[1])

When Rene Descartes wrote these very famous words in 1644 the key point was — if I can think, I must exist. That this phrase gets used so very often in so many different situations speaks to how important the act of thinking is to who we are and how we exist in the world.

So thinking is important, but further to this *how* we think is important and influences how we feel and act in response to what goes on around us.

Imagine this scenario:

> You wake up and get ready for work, go down to the car driveway and the car is not there! Someone must have stolen it! You start to panic, you keep the fuel card in the car, and whoever has the car can go anywhere. Your whole week will be ruined; you had a weekend planned

---

[1] Originally written in French, but later translated into Latin, the phrase includes 'doubt', with the idea being that if you can doubt your existence and are able to think about this you must therefore exist.

away with your partner, and a big meeting at work this morning that you will be late for. Your boss will be furious. You can feel your heart racing and you feel sick in the stomach. Why do bad things always happen to me? You run inside to call the police and then your partner reminds you that you caught the bus home yesterday and left the car at work.

How often have you hit the panic button only to find your worse fear was not true or did not happen?

Most of the time we think in an automatic way, without effort, and in patterns we have learned and practiced all our lives. How many times have you reflected that someone you know (or maybe even you) always thinks the worst, or the best, or jumps to conclusions? It matters, because we do tend to respond as if our thoughts are absolutely true, and if our mind perceives a tiger out there our bodies will react as if there really is one and will set off the physical stress response accordingly. You can test this out for yourself in the following simple thinking exercise.

First, think about something that happened in the past that was really upsetting. Remind yourself where this was, who was there and think about what happened and what was said. Think and remember what happened. How do you feel right now after thinking about this?

Now think about something that you would really like to happen, something you have dreamed about. Who would be there with you and where would you be? What feelings do these thoughts and images bring up in you in this moment?

For both of these exercises the reality of who and where you are right now didn't change, but how you feel probably did. The only thing that did change was what you were thinking about. How we think and what we think about affects how we feel.

Thinking Patterns

We learn as we grow up how to think and be in the world. If the main message we received was that the world is not a safe place, or that we are not worthwhile, then the way we think and react may be to be hyper vigilant for danger or to tend to blame ourselves or feel guilty when things go wrong.

On the other hand, if we were mostly led to believe that by and large things will be okay in the long run and that we are competent and able to surmount most things, we might be less likely to jump to the worst possible conclusions.

However you think or react to situations, this is not about saying one way is better or worse. However, if you predict or assume the worse most or much of the time, this is not only upsetting but also exhausting!

There are some common thinking patterns people use that just don't help when you are in a stressful situation.

- *Catastrophising*. Thinking of the worst possible outcome that could happen
- *Black and White Thinking* (also called 'all or nothing thinking' or 'my way or the highway'). Thinking that things have to go a certain way or it will be a complete disaster.
- *Self- blame*. Think that it is all your fault
- *Overgeneralising*. Taking one event and turning it into a sweeping generalisation about how things will always be
- *The Negative Mental Filter*. Seeing only the negative aspects of a situation and ignoring all of the positives
- *Jumping to Conclusions*. Assuming something is negative when there is actually not much evidence to support it.

The trouble with these patterns of thinking is that they can lead you to feel anxious or depressed and that they don't lead you to generate other possibilities or help you look at things in a balanced way. They are pretty much 'dead end' thinking. And they can also keep you awake late at night when all is quiet and there is nothing to distract you from thinking the worst.

A Different Approach

A different approach is to pick up the habit of checking your thinking for distortion. (Now don't go overboard on this, there is such a thing as too much introspection!) When you notice yourself feeling down or on edge or angry, ask yourself — 'What am I thinking about to make me feel this way?' Secondly, ask yourself — 'Is my way of thinking about my current situation helping me or hindering me? Is this a typical way that I react to situations?' This is the first step. Then, if you do identify unhelpful thoughts that are recurring or causing you to worry more, then challenge them. Say to yourself — 'How true is this thought really and how helpful is this thought to me? Is there a better way for me to think about this? What would my best friend, or someone I really respect, say to me if they could read my thoughts?'

A good example of the above approach would be if you find yourself thinking something along the lines of 'I am not going to initiate sex with my partner because it won't work and then they will think I am worthless as a mate'. This is a combination of catastrophising and all-or-nothing thinking. Another example is recollecting all of the times that your partner seemed tired or got cross with you over the week and thinking 'They are not coping and it is all my fault'. This is a combination of using a negative mental filter and jumping to conclusions.

You could start to challenge this thinking by reminding yourself of all the things about each other that you both value outside of sex, such as companionship and family ties. You could also remember that you know sex after prostate cancer takes time and patience and effort, and that this is not your fault or anyone else's. (Get the idea?)

Thinking as Processing

However, all of this does not mean you should never have a negative thought. This would be ridiculous. Negative thoughts about your cancer can't physically hurt you, they are just thoughts and they don't make your cancer worse, just in case anyone has thrown that old chestnut at you. There is no evidence to support the idea that negative thoughts about cancer make the cancer worse.

It is normal for people to, at times, have what we call 'intrusive thoughts' about their cancer. These are unwanted negative thoughts about the cancer that just pop into your head often when you least expect it. These thoughts are most likely just normal mental processing of what is for anyone a 'big deal' life issue. In other words, this is a normal and necessary part of coming to terms with cancer and accepting this as now part of your life history. Trying desperately to never think a negative thought or to even think at all about the cancer (this is given the fancy name of 'cognitive or thought avoidance') increases the likelihood that that thought will continue to pop up and cause even more distress.

Intrusive negative thoughts are really only a problem if they are driving ongoing strong feelings of distress, or are getting in the way of you having a happy life. It doesn't help you if the minute you get a negative thought about the cancer you beat yourself up about it. Remember, they are just thoughts.

Another approach with negative thoughts is to notice they are there, perhaps even label the thought —'Ah Ah! There I go again, thinking that it is all my fault that my partner is tired' and then deliberately shift your focus elsewhere to where you are right now in this very moment. In brief, leave the past and the future to worry about themselves. Live for the now and in the present moment — stop to smell the roses.

Activity

For the next week, keep notes in your journal of the times when you find yourself feeling more upset or stressed. Jot down the day and time, where you are and who you are with, what is going on and most importantly what you are thinking and feeling.

After a week of keeping these notes, take some time to look them over and see if you can identify a pattern. Do you have a typical way of thinking that you can identify? Are there any of the negative common thinking patterns mentioned above. Are your thoughts realistic or based on accurate or true and known information? Are these thoughts helping or hindering you? Is there a way you could think about what is happening that would serve you better?

Talk this over if you can with your partner or a close and trusted friend. Ask them to support you in coming up with more helpful view of what is going on. If you don't feel you can talk about these thoughts with someone else, or just prefer not to, become your own best friend. Write down a different way to look at the problem or challenge you are facing that expresses kindness and care to yourself.

Now, find some time in the next week to sit in the garden or go for a short walk. As you do this notice what is around you. Focus your attention on the finer details of the trees or plants, how the wind plays with your surroundings, and how the sunlight falls and changes the colours around you. Are there small animals you notice, ants or lizards? What noises can you hear? Is there traffic in the distance, can you hear laughter in the background, and the sounds of your own breathing? Now notice how you feel. Practice using this grounding technique next time that you notice getting carried away with negative thoughts.

Personal Stories

Below is a personal story from a different David about his prostate cancer experience and how he has learnt to manage worrying thoughts and keep stress under control.

David

I was diagnosed in 1999 and had a radical prostatectomy in 2000. It was a pretty tough time, and while I had a great surgeon technically, his communication skills could have been better! I had the idea that I had to have the surgery as quickly as possible or the cancer would kill me and my 'head space' was exploding! I know now that that wasn't actually the case, I wasn't on death's door, and I could have taken my time a little more.

The main problems I had after surgery were urinary continence and impotence. At the time the urinary continence was my biggest concern. Back then I wasn't in touch with a support group, and so this meant I had to search out information for myself, with not much help to be honest. I looked on the internet, read books, and then got myself to a physiotherapist to learn pelvic floor exercises, and over time, about twelve months, the problem resolved. My GP was a help as well.

A challenge here was managing my thinking. I have always had a tendency to worry. My mother was like this and I think I learnt this way of thinking from her. I guess I am a natural worrier! All those 'what ifs?' scare the hell out of you. 'What if I never get my urine control back and I have to wear pads for the rest of my life? What if people I know see me buying incontinence pads? What if it gets worse? What if I leak in public?' You can really get into a dark place psychologically if you let these types of thoughts take over.

The way I have taught myself to manage this is first to notice and be more aware of my thinking patterns. None of this comes naturally to me, I have had to learn to do this. Even after all these years I still do keep an eye on myself for this because worries about the cancer do come back from time to time. When I notice I am doing negative 'what if' type of thinking, I tell myself to stop it and either distract myself by reading a good thriller (great for distraction!) or do something physical like wash the car or walk the dog. Sometimes I just change the subject in my head or change the thought by rationalising. I tell myself that the worrying thought just isn't true and I try and talk to myself in a more positive way. Kind of remind myself that none of this is the end of the world, hard things happen in life and that is just the way of it. I guess I now see having had prostate cancer in that way, as a phase of life I have been through. I do believe that you are in charge of your own destiny, there is no good fairy flitting around to fix things for you, if you want it fixed you need to do it yourself.

I moved cities after my cancer. Having cancer made me reassess how I was living and I decided I wanted less stress and a better quality of life. Cancer made me really realise I was not going to live forever and it was like a little light switched on in my head. My priorities changed, and work didn't seem like the main game anymore. It was a good move for me.

I have always been pretty curious about life and open to what it has to teach me. I am pretty lucky to have a great family, good friends, and I make sure that I keep connected to them, that helps as well. My friends and family are my anchor. When I retired that was tough as well. I was bored and cranky, irritable and angry a fair bit of the time. Not much fun to be around. I worked it out though, did some part time work for a while and tried different things. It was a big transition. I volunteer now and run a prostate cancer support group and I feel like this is a really worthwhile thing to do. It is still hard for many men to find support when they need it and our group helps them see that prostate cancer is not the end of everything. Blokes often come to our group pretty downcast, but after seeing other men doing well they feel reassured and becoming better informed makes the lights really go on!

■ ■ ■ ■

De-Stressing: How to Look After Yourself and Keep Well

It is probably fair to say that many of us spend a lot of time and energy working, looking after family, getting jobs done, keeping house, and not much time (or enough time) taking care of our health. How many times have you either told yourself, or been given advice from others, that you need to relax more, take time out to de-stress, exercise more regularly, and eat better? It is easy to brush this off as a nice idea but one that will need to wait until later — when things settle down, are less busy and you can finally find that time for yourself.

I suspect most of us think this way. The problem however is that this is a delaying tactic. You might never get around to the task of looking after yourself in this way, and so you just keep on 'keeping on' and getting a little more tired, tense, and less at your best as time goes on. The time to look after your health will never be right unless you claim it and make it so. So do it now!

Why bother? Because letting physical and mental tension build up without a break is like driving your car or motorbike at full throttle all day, every day, no matter what the circumstances. The outcome of this (at least in a motor vehicle) is that the engine wears quickly, the brakes will soon lose their effectiveness, you go through too much petrol, and eventually the thing just stops, or even worse you lose control. You would not treat your car this way so why do this to your body?

Looking after your physical and mental well-being is important for everyone, but especially important if you are going through the stressful experience of either being diagnosed with cancer or supporting someone who has cancer.

The first aim then in looking after yourself is to reduce *physical tension* in your body. Think back to the earlier chapter in this book that overviewed the stress response. When you are under pressure and in a situation of threat your body reacts by pumping itself up with action hormones (the 'flight or fight' response) that create physical tension. Not only is this unpleasant to experience but if it goes on unchecked it is not good for your overall health. So there is a very good pragmatic reason to use strategies or tools to reduce unwanted or unnecessary physical body tension.

The second aim, and this is just as important, is to reduce *mental tension* and try to clear your mind of worrying thoughts at least some of the time. Mental tension can drive or increase physical tension in a reinforcing cycle, so you need to target both aspects.

There are lots of ways to relax — if you google relaxation techniques (the last time I checked) you will get over five million hits! You will have you own usual ways of relaxing, and this might include reading, watching movies, playing golf or bowls, dancing or socialising. If you have let these activities slip in the 'busy-ness' of coping with the cancer, or life in general, then now is a good time to get back on track. Make time in your schedule for doing the things that you enjoy and find relaxing. As well though, you might consider learning some new skills or taking on some new activities that are specifically about reducing tension and looking after your physical and mental well-being.

Learning to Relax — Practice makes Perfect

With all dedicated relaxation techniques it is a good idea to practice them first in a private and quiet place where you won't get disturbed, and in comfortable clothes. As well, don't wait until you are stressed and tense to give it a go. Try it out when you already feel pretty calm until you get the hang of it. Learning relaxation techniques is in some ways like learning to ride a bicycle for the first time — if feels strange and you are not sure if you are getting it right until suddenly you get an 'Ah-Ha' moment, your body and mind puts it all together, and it starts to feel like second nature. So keep the trainer wheels and practice regularly while you learn how to control your body and mind in this way. Once you get more experienced and skilful you will find that you are able to more effortlessly apply these strategies when you need them the most.

Take a Breath

Controlling and slowing your breath is a very simple way to calm your body. Breathing techniques are easy to do anywhere and anytime, and because they are not obvious to those around you they can be done in almost any situation of stress and you won't look weird!

As a first step, find a comfortable and quiet place to sit and focus for a few minutes on being aware of your breathing. Notice how the breath moves in and out of your nose and chest, and how your chest muscles contract and relax as you breathe. Listen to the sound of your breath as you breathe in and out. Be aware of your posture and of how your shoulders sit as you breathe. If your shoulders are tight and hunched drop them down on your out-breath.

Next, count slowly to four in every *in* and *out* breath you take. Focus your mind on the count, and breathe in a slow and relaxed and comfortable way in time to the count. Do this for several minutes as your body gets used to slow and controlled breathing.

Now stop and notice how you feel. This is a quick and easy de-stress strategy that can be easily applied to good effect when stuck in traffic, waiting in a doctor's office for a check-up, or at night just before you go to sleep to relax yourself down.

This exercise can be extended by adding in at the end, for a few breaths only, holding your breath for a count of two. You can also add visualisation or imagery by focussing your mind on a safe and relaxing scenario or image towards the end of the exercise, once your breathing has slowed down. This might mean building a picture in your mind of a relaxing place and activity, such as swimming in the sea or walking in a forest, and imagining the colours and sounds and physical sensations you would experience if you were there.

There are of course other techniques you might try, such as progressive relaxation as one example. This approach is where you progressively tense and relax different areas of your body, often starting at the toes and working your way up. The best thing about breathing exercises, and why I tend to teach these first, is that in my experience most people can get the hang of it and get a good effect pretty quickly. If you would like to really broaden your skills in this though, you might also want to try meditation techniques.

Meditation and Mindfulness

Meditation originated thousands of years ago and can be described as an approach to life and people that encompasses acceptance, self-knowledge and awareness, love free from expectation, 'letting go' or non-attachment, and at a higher level the search for enlightenment.

Meditation techniques are the central tool in the Buddhist tool box for life, and these focus on calming the mind. The purpose generally speaking is to gain a deeper sense of awareness of the self and the world through stilling the mind. This leads to improved well-being and a greater resilience to challenges and the problems life can throw at you.

More recently some of these ideas have been packaged as 'mindfulness' where the focus is deliberately paying attention to the present moment, or moment-by-moment awareness without judgement, in a way that leads to a better ability to manage thoughts and feelings.

It might sound a little vague, but there is good evidence that mindfulness and related meditation approaches can improve well-being, so it is well worth considering and trying out. As with all relaxation techniques it does tend to be 'horses for courses'. What suits one person may not suit another — it is a very individual thing. However, being open to these ideas and what they might bring for you is another good way of being your own best friend.

Try this quick mindfulness exercise and see how you go!

Find a place in the garden or a quiet room where you can sit comfortably and uninterrupted for about ten minutes. The goal of this exercise is to stop and become aware of your physical location and your surroundings sense-by-sense. Before you start, check your watch.

First, become aware of how you feel now that you have stopped what you were doing. What thoughts — or echoes of thoughts — have you carried with you into this moment and what feelings are here now? Perhaps scan your body and notice if there are any points of tightness or tension in your body. Next — deliberately gather your attention and redirect it to the feeling of your breath as it enters, and then again, as it leaves your body. Do this for several breaths — almost as if you are dropping anchor into this moment using your breath. Now expand your awareness around your breath and begin to notice how you feel physically in this space. Are you cool or warm? Feel the bottom of your feet and how your feet feel against the ground. Are you sitting firmly? How does your backside feel against the chair? Your back?

Listen to the sounds around you. What can you hear in the background? Road noise? Birds? The sound of your breathing? Choose one sound and try to notice the details of the sound — the volume, the pitch, the gaps between the sounds. Notice if your mind starts to tell you stories about what you can hear, and, as best you can bring your mind back to focus on the details of the sounds themselves.

Now look around you and find a visual focus point, it might be a plant leaf or a photograph on the wall and closely notice the details of this point. Notice the shades of colour, the texture, the shape — how the sun falls on this spot. Maintain this focus as long as you can and try and notice the details that you might not have seen before.

95

Now, check your watch again. How long were you able to keep this up for? Three minutes? Five? It can be surprisingly hard to stop for ten minutes and become aware of our surroundings. How did you feel while you were doing this exercise? What was the state of your mind? Did you feel frustrated at being still or did you feel a sense of calm?

This focussing activity is just one example of the type of techniques that you might work on to master meditation. I have found that it does help in a wide range of situations where drawing your attention to the details of your surroundings can distract you from irritation, boredom or even pain. At the very least it can help you to become more aware of what is on your mind and how you are feeling physically — and take you away from your automatic train of thought — if only for a few moments. Meditation does take training and practice though, however if you are interested in learning more there are excellent books and courses around to get you started, and there are a few listed in the Appendix. I recommend having a go!

Exercise

For many men exercise is their preferred way to reduce physical and mental stress. They feel comfortable with the approach and indeed exercise is generally associated with better psychological well-being.

However, there are many other good reasons to exercise if you have had a diagnosis of cancer or are close to someone who has. First, there is evidence that physical inactivity and being overweight are risk factors for not only getting some cancers but also doing less well after the cancer with regards to quality of life and cancer recurrence. Second, many men who have prostate cancer are also at risk for heart or cardiovascular disease due to their age, as are their partners. So reducing your risk of other chronic diseases so you can enjoy your life together in good health makes sense.

Even better, exercise can help reduce some of the negative effects of prostate cancer treatment, such as muscle and bone loss from hormone blocking drugs. Further on in the list of beneficial effects, exercise can improve urinary control and sexual function, reduce fatigue and tiredness, improve sleep, help with balance and reduce the risk of falls, and is associated with better thinking (cognitive ability) — all important things for enjoying a full and satisfying life after prostate cancer.

Of course, we all know we should exercise more. The trouble is getting motivated to start, finding the time, choosing a way to exercise that you can practically stick to, and then keeping it up. A good way to start is to first think about how much you value your health and well-being and the things you are looking forward to in the future that you want to be physically well for. From this you need to set goals for physical activity that match what matters most to you, and then make a commitment to do this for *yourself*.

Key practical steps to exercise are to have a health check-up with your doctor before you take on a new exercise plan, and then get really good advice from an expert (such as an exercise physiologist) to make sure that the plan you have will get you where you want to go. Unguided exercise can be pretty hit and miss in terms of achieving results, and without good advice you are more likely to end with a strain or over-use injury that slows you down. In a way, what you want is the maximum benefit for the least effort — an efficient and targeted exercise plan that gets you where you want to go.

There are two different types of exercise you will want to aim for: strengthening (or resistance) exercise and aerobic exercise. Resistance exercise, using as examples weights or elastic bands, will build muscle and muscle strength where you need and want it most. Aerobic exercise will build your cardiovascular fitness and help with weight control. Getting a good balance of these two approaches will keep your body working at its best and also help keep you free from injuries. As a general rule you need to exercise for twenty to sixty minutes at least three times a week to get results. Higher intensity exercise is now seen as a very effective means of improving cardiovascular fitness. In practical terms, this involves exercising with a higher heart rate but perhaps for shorter periods (separated by 'recovery' bouts of lower intensity exercise).

The final point to make is that it can be easier to stick to an exercise plan if you have a friend or partners to exercise with. It just makes it more fun! As well, if you set exercise goals and share these with a friend or your partner they can support and help motivate you to keep it up.

Activity

If you already meditate three days a week and are currently training to climb Kilimanjaro, then no activity work for you! On the other hand, if you are like most people and could do with a little less tension and a little more exercise, you need to set some goals.

Think about how you feel most of the time, do you think you have room for improvement in the way you look after yourself? Use the checklist below as a start and prioritise which of these things you would most like to work on.

- Exercising more

- Feeling more calm

- Reducing my weight

- Feeling stronger physically

- Any other ways?

The next step is to draw up a plan of attack. Be clear about your goals first and the short and medium term milestones you want to reach, and when you expect to get there. List the steps you will need to take to move towards these milestones, who and what you need to help you achieve these, and what barriers you might need to cross or deal with as you go. Consider that there are many different ways to help you achieve your goals. You might like to join a yoga or tai chi class, start walking with a friend, or just make some quiet space in each day to 'drop anchor' and calm your mind. Finally, pick a date to get started, tell your close friends or partners about your plan so they can keep a check on you, and go for it!

Remember, set backs are normal, and watch yourself for unhelpful 'all or nothing' thinking. Most things that are worthwhile are effort, but if you never start you most certainly will not get there.

Personal Stories

Below is a personal story from Charles about how he came to take up an exercise program to help with prostate cancer treatment side effects that has turned into a normal way of life for him and his partner. Jan and Gordon talk about how they use mindfulness and breathing techniques to manage stress. Finally, Roger talks about how he got into dragon boating and how this has enhanced his fitness and his social life!

Charles

I was diagnosed with an aggressive prostate cancer in 2011. I was 76 years of age at the time. Because of my age and also that I had had heart surgery in the past, my urologist and radiation oncologist suggested radiation therapy, both brachytherapy and external beam, and a six-month course of hormone blocking injections. It was a big shock at the time, and I do think that is the biggest challenge, getting over that shock. In the end though, what can you do but take a positive outlook? I just thought: 'Alright then, I can't change it, so I will do my best to fix it and do what I can to get well'.

The side effects of the hormone treatment were pretty tough. I put weight on around my girth, and that bothered me since I had always kept my weight steady. The hot flushes were the worse, five or six a night, and in the summer heat in the west that is hard going. It gave me new sympathy for what women go through in the menopause! The best tip I got was when my doctor referred me to an exercise program based at Edith Cowan University at their Health and Wellness Institute in Perth. I went along there and was assessed by the exercise physiology team, they looked at my bone density, my physical fitness, a really comprehensive check-up. From that they worked out an exercise program suited to my individual needs. The program they set me went for three months initially, it was in a small group of three people, and included walking on a treadmill as well as a series of exercises involving weights. Things like lifting leg weights, step ups, and shoulder and arm resistance exercises. We had to tinker with the program now and again though. I have arthritis and after a while I just couldn't manage the dumbbells. The alternative we tried was a medicine ball and that was terrific and enabled me to keep up my upper body exercises. Whenever there was a problem the exercise physiologist found a creative way to get round it. Once my plan was sorted out I was able to do the exercise program in my local gymnasium to cut down my travel, as I live in Freemantle. After six weeks I went back to Edith Cowan to have the tests again and to check my progress and everything was improved! My bone density was better, my muscles had tightened up again and I was much stronger. In fact, by the end of three months I had improved an old back injury to the point where I didn't need a walking stick anymore, so I was better than ever.

Apart from the physical benefits of the exercise program, I think it helps you mentally to be able to do something to help yourself. We did the program in a small group, so I made new friends, and the gymnasium is a pretty stimulating environment, lots of people to talk to and lots going on. It got me out of the house as well and really established clearly to me that I was not the only one going through this. That helped a lot.

I have kept the exercise up even though I am now not on the hormone treatment. My wife has always been very supportive, we have been married now for 57 years, and she wanted to get involved as well. So we bought ourselves a treadmill and an exercise bike and some weights and we now do the routine at home, every day. It is pretty simple really. We also try and walk about two to three kilometres a day. You do have to be disciplined to keep it up, but it helps to do it together and the benefits are well worth it. To keep well, this is one thing I can do.

Gordon

One of the hardest things I find is trying not to spend too much energy worrying about what might happen tomorrow.

My view is we need to live for today but we also have to live with the understanding of the disease, which the doctors tell me is at the stage where I can't be cured. Knowing that makes a big difference to what you are doing. At the moment everything is fine, the path I am on right now is that I can do basically whatever I like and still enjoy it. There are times though when the thoughts come in, like when the Olympic games finished, is that the last Olympic games I will be able to watch? When those thoughts come in I get some sense of urgency, like I need to do this now because I might not be able to do in the future. It's a case of also being aware of the situation I am in and asking myself if what I am doing has a point, or should I invest my energy elsewhere? Jan says I am a great procrastinator, she calls me 'Random Global' — I have a picture with 4000 things in it that I want to do, and prioritising these is hard! There are so many things out there to do, you move forward a little bit on this one and a little bit on that one, and some things get to completion and others don't. That's probably the frustrating part for me is that I don't complete as many things as I should. But that doesn't stop me trying.

For de-stressing, the thing that is best for me at the moment is the breathing exercise. When I get into a situation that feels a bit tough, I do a two minute breathing exercise, which is just a relaxation approach. I also try and focus on the now, the present, focus on what I am doing and move everything else away. When I get aches and pains or when a situation develops and I am starting to feel stressed, I focus on what I am doing now, the very simple things, and what I am doing in this moment. It helps me to keep going and come out the other side in a positive state. I find the relaxation tapes help as well, being able to sit and listen and take your mind away. I really enjoy doing that although haven't been doing this lately as much as I should.

Jan

I found out about mindfulness from a counsellor I was seeing at the Cancer Council Queensland. She mentioned that this course was coming up and asked would I be interested. It was an eight week group course, I mentioned it to Gordon and asked if he wanted to come to, and he said why not, so that is how we got in.

For the first few weeks it was difficult. I guess I was concerned that Gordon was the only bloke in the room, in fact I was quite concerned and distressed for his sake. I could only imagine how I would have felt if I had been the only woman in a room full of men, so there was that to it. But he settled in about half way through the course. By that stage it was almost genderless; there was only the odd occasion when we would roll our eyes at each other! The other thing we did was to make sure that after every mindfulness course we would go to dinner somewhere in town to some bohemian restaurant, so we always had something to look forward to afterwards. As it turned out, while we always enjoyed our dinners, we didn't really need to go dinner afterwards because the sessions became more and more enjoyable. We began to really look forward them. They were difficult in the first instance because the actual act of mindfulness is really hard at the start. All of us in the group were struggling. I guess what I am saying is that mindfulness is not an easy practice to learn after many, many years of letting your brain do whatever it wants to do, whenever it wants to do it. Probably up to week five it was a real struggle, after that I stopped judging myself, and then it became a more enjoyable process.

The mindfulness exercise which I find the easiest is the one where I do part body scan, part listening and part feeling. For me to do fifty minutes of just scanning my body is torture and I find it really difficult. It is much easier for me to listen to what's going on outside and just enjoy the simple things like the sun on your body or the sounds around you.

Roger

I was diagnosed with prostate cancer just over nine years ago, which was pretty traumatic at the time. I had a great surgeon though, and he got me through it really. Then, about one year later my PSA started to rise, I went on hormone blocking treatment, but again after about another year later the problem recurred again. Luckily, there was a clinical trial, a vaccine trial actually, that my doctor found I was eligible for. Since then, between the trial and my hormonal therapy, I have kept really well.

One thing I do for myself is keep very active. About four years ago I got into dragon boating. Dragon boating is great exercise, you actually use your stomach muscle or core strength more than your arms, and I can tell you that working out in a dragon boat four times a week gets you fit! I have always loved the water. When I was a baby my grandpa used to take me out netting for flounder, and I would play with the baby flounder in the bottom of the boat! I grew up in Hobart and was always on the water, fishing on the jetty, and rowing dinghies and sailing yachts on the Derwent River. So when a friend suggested dragon boating to me, it was a great fit. You also get to meet a lot of great people, from all walks of life, so from a social point of view it is brilliant as well as fun. There is also something really

105

calming about being close to the water, a great mix.

About the time I took up dragon boating I also decided to improve my diet, moving to more fresh fruit and vegetables. Over time I lost 20 kilograms in weight, so now I am a healthy weight for my height and age. The exercise also helps with the muscle wastage that you get from the hormone treatment, and the tiredness.

I do a lot of volunteering as well, and a lot of this is connected to exercise. I have been working with the Relay for Life program of the Cancer Council Queensland for many years, and in fact in 2010 I was named the Relay for Life International Hero of Hope, one of only 13 at that time in the world. Relay for Life is a fund raising event that involves walking or running for 24 hours in teams. My aim now is to raise money with the hope I can save more than one life from cancer. This is all I do with my life now and I enjoy all the people I am involved with. I have the normal side effects from the hormone treatment, mostly tiredness and a bit of a dull head at times. I am used to these effects now and my way of coping is to keep busy, look after my overall wellness, and not pay these negative effects too much attention. I will be 70 this year and I am still standing up and enjoying life so I can't complain!

■ ■ ■ ■

Solving Problems After Treatment

So, back to 'facing the tiger': If I can't fight or run, what can I do? Adopting a problem solving approach is one good option.

Problem solving is of course part of everyday life, we do it all the time often with little focused thought. Some people are more efficient at solving problems than others, but most of us could probably do better at this with a more planned approach. After a prostate cancer diagnosis most men and their partners will at one time or another run into problems they haven't dealt with before. This is very unfamiliar territory for most people and it can feel a little overwhelming.

In this situation using a more systematic approach to solving problems can help. In brief, this approach breaks the problem down into manageable chunks and helps you move forward towards an answer. A problem solving approach can be applied to very practical problems, like coping with treatment side effects, and also for emotional or relationship problems that are sometimes a bit harder to talk about or deal with straight up.

The first step is to be clear about what the problem is, so define the problem and find accurate information about the issue so that you understand why it has arisen and what it means. This might mean reading over cancer treatment booklets from a reputable source such as Prostate Cancer Foundation of Australia or the Cancer Council, talking to your doctor or prostate care nurse, and meeting with and talking to other men who have also had prostate cancer or their partners who might have experienced this problem and be able to provide advice from a personal perspective.

From this you will be able to generate different options or possibilities for dealing with the problem. The more alternative solutions you generate the better. The point is to come up with as many different ideas as possible.

Next, evaluate the pros and cons of each possible solution. This should include what help you might need and from whom, how confident you feel about each approach working for you, and from this a preferred option should emerge.

Once you have a preferred option, then you can start on the plan. Your plan needs to be clear about the steps you will need to take, and should have a timeline for each step. Finally, be clear about what success would mean for this problem and how you will evaluate for yourself how you have gone. As you go though, be prepared to re-evaluate your plan and adjust or change it if it doesn't seem to be working for you. Having a flexible approach is crucial.

Here is one example of how this approach could be applied to a problem that is not unusual after prostate cancer treatment.

Example: Solving Urinary Problems

Bill and Hillary are a couple from Sydney in their early sixties and they have been married for 15 years. Bill had a radical prostatectomy eight weeks ago and is still having problems with urinary control. He is wearing a pad all the time, and during the day has to change this at least three times. As a result he is not going out of the house much, his partner Hillary is irritable about them staying home all of the time, and Bill is feeling frustrated with the pace of his recovery. Because of the urinary leakage they haven't tried to have sex and both Bill and Hillary find it hard to talk about this.

If you reflect on what is happening for Bill and Hillary there are actually *at least* six pieces or 'chunks' to this problem:

- Urinary leakage
- Being housebound
- Feeling stressed about recovering from treatment
- Not feeling close as a couple

- Not having sex
- Having difficulty communicating

It is important to be clear about all the chunks in this problem, because although they all seem related, each of these issues need different strategies and all involve both Bill and Hillary. Fortunately, Bill and Hillary eventually decide they need to use a problem solving approach to move forward.

Considering each of these issues they decide to start with urinary leakage. By reading up on the subject and talking to Bill's surgeon they know that the reason this can happen is damage at the time of surgery to the tissues and nerves that control passing urine. Understanding that this is a problem that usually resolves over time helps, and knowing that if Bill does regular pelvic floor muscles he can speed up the repair process, provides a basis for a plan. Bill decides to go to a physiotherapist to get help with learning how to do pelvic floor exercises and Hillary decides she needs to learn them as well. Since the babies and the menopause her urine control has not been great either!

Bill goes to a local prostate cancer support group meeting and he is able to borrow a copy of a self-help book on pelvic floor exercises from a chap he meets there. At the support group Bill meets other men who have also experienced this problem and he learns that it is pretty common to be still using a few pads a day at this stage. He is reassured to find out that he will probably be down to one pad a day in a month or so and that most men are dry by six months. The men he talks to also have great practical tips for managing this problem when out and about. He now feels less like he is the only one with this problem and more hopeful about the future. It is a relief! He has found a map of where the public toilets are in the city centre and he feels confident enough to make a plan with Hillary to go to the movies together next weekend.

Hillary and Bill decide to make a time to talk about how they are coping as a couple. They set aside a morning and share with each other how they have been feeling of late. Both Hillary and Bill agree they want to get back to being closer and more like they were before the cancer. As a first step they agree that more hugs and touching and physical closeness, but with no expectation of sex, is needed. Bill wants to get his urine control a bit better before they try at sex, even though they both know that urine leakage during sex is not at all harmful. They do want to get sex back on track in the future though, so Bill makes an appointment with his doctor for both him and Hillary to find out about what options are available for helping Bill get an erection. Both Bill and Hillary are aware that working on Bill having regular erections earlier rather than later is part of good 'penis health' after prostate cancer treatment.

In the meantime Hillary books a weekend away at the beach for her and Bill, and buys an erotic book and some massage oil, just in case they get in the mood for some extra closeness. The main plan though includes long walks on the beach and relaxation. Hillary has been doing some meditation classes to help her relax and de-stress and Bill has agreed to give it a go (or at least try the breath control exercises) while they are on their weekend away.

■■■■

If you look over this hypothetical story (although I have known many men and their partners who have experienced these actual problems) you can see that each chunk of the problem needed different strategies, even though the issues were all related and seemed to stem from the urinary problems. Bill and Hillary took the time first to be clear about the problem and talk about it together. Their next step was to get more information about what they could do about it and then to talk this through to develop an agreed preferred approach. They now will need to put this into action, and if needed revise the plan as they go along.

Taking your time with a well-considered plan will help you to not miss important opportunities to make things work better for you. Involving your partner or a support person, like a son or daughter or close friend, in the making of the plan will help make sure you are both pulling together and working as a team.

Activity

> In your note pad or journal make a list of the main problems that are worrying you right now. Do this separately on your own and then share these with your partner. Do you have some problems that you both are concerned about and could work on together? Are there things worrying your partner that you were unaware of?
>
> Next, prioritise this list using number 1 for the problem that is most important to you right now, 2 for the next most important, and so on.
>
> Pick off your top three priorities and ask yourself if you understand clearly how this problem has arisen. If you need more information about the problem make a decision to find out more.
>
> Once you feel you are well informed generate a list of possible actions you could take to help with each priority and consider which actions you feel comfortable doing and most confident about. Think about who can help you with this and what extra support you might need, and what milestones you want to reach and when.
>
> Now you have a plan you can move into action, but remember that if all does not go the way you planned or hoped it is okay to re-consider and revise the plan.

Personal Stories

Below is a personal story from Norman about how he approached problems he faced after prostate cancer treatment, and this included getting outside support with the help of his son Tristan, when things got very tough. Gerry talks about how he was bit too chilled out after treatment and Graham shares how a very tough time turned around once he got the right advice.

Norman

Being diagnosed in late 2007 was a real shock. The prognosis was challenging and required a different approach to treatment. The best option was considered to be brachytherapy, followed by external beam radiotherapy, and hormone treatment for a few months before the brachytherapy. The hormone therapy was awful, it brings about a huge loss of energy, and makes working accurately challenging. Simply going for a walk was difficult. The hot flushes happened any time and could be embarrassing. I knew I had to try to understand this cancer and the treatment to make some sense of it all, and thereby accept and know what lay ahead. This I did using many sources such as the Internet, discussion with health professionals, and contact with the Brisbane Prostate Cancer Support Group. Gradually I felt I had built a picture that reassured me.

The big day arrived, and I was very confident that the next two parts of the treatment would be a breeze. I knew all about this stuff! In fact the brachytherapy went very well, really just as expected. There are a few things that are confronting, as with any surgery. A few days after the brachytherapy I started daily external beam radiation. At first this seemed to go well, until my mind started to 'spin out' with thoughts of radiation burn, accuracy of the beam, the challenge to my masculinity, and the thought that I may die before my wife.

I was still at work, so medical appointments were either early morning or late afternoon. You need to have a full bladder for each treatment. This added to my desperation until my wife suggested timing the start of hydration to arrive on the treatment table full, and bursting, but avoiding accidents. I always needed a pit stop afterwards and still had the occasional accident on the table. Even though the treatment staff told me 'Mate that's all part of it, happens all the time, don't worry about it' I did worry about it! I was not coping with things and I needed help. I took time off work, as that had become difficult. My iPod was loaded with calming music to help me relax before and during treatment. I changed appointments to mid morning or mid afternoon. These changes gave slight relief, but the issues were getting harder to avoid.

My son Tristan had been making sure that everything was going well, but from the background. He could see that things were difficult for me, which impacted on my wife's concerns, as she was driving me to many appointments, and making sure I was progressing. He picked up on the fact that I needed some outside help to try to calm down and make sense of things. My son has always been very supportive of both of us. He never tries to run the show. Rather, he will look at situations and gently suggest some ideas. He believes in getting the right help and find out how to source it. One of his friends knew a psychologist with a practice close to us. Between the two of them getting things happening, I had a very rewarding time making some sense out of my anxiety and somewhat irrational thoughts. This continued for a period with another counsellor. While it is hard to sit down with a complete stranger and lay out your innermost issues it becomes less so as you work through what you choose to change, and is in fact very rewarding.

My son and I have become much closer in recent times, in terms of expressing appreciation and love for one another. Once he had reached sixteen such things seemed past history. But now a good man hug and a brush cheek kiss is so welcome for both of us.

I have learnt a lot from my cancer journey. I have changed the way I live, interact with others, and now enjoy every moment of my life. Learning to meditate to calm the body, mind and soul is satisfying. Living in the moment, savouring what is happening right now is my aim. While not always easy, sitting having coffee in a sunny spot, hearing the birds, feeling a slight breeze, or the smell of a freshly baked cookie grabs me now. Just as does the crackle of an open fire on a winter night, the smell of a barbecue, happy conversation and the clinking of glasses, and time with friends.

It is important to respect yourself, and have the courage to be yourself. Life throws some unpleasant things at us. At dark times, take a tool which you have in your tool belt, apply it and surprise yourself.

Tristan

I couldn't believe it when Dad was diagnosed with prostate cancer. It didn't seem fair. Mum and Dad approached Dad's diagnosis as a team, and Dad initially approached the whole situation with calm confidence. He seemed confident in the treatment and in his medical team, and he even laughed off some of the more unpleasant aspects of the Brachytherapy treatment — including what we referred to as the porcupine stage!

It all changed when Dad started hormone therapy and radiotherapy. The confidence vanished, and was replaced with fatigue, doubt and increasing despair. At first I thought it was a side effect of the hormone treatment. He was depressed, and was obsessing about his treatment. Then Dad refused to attend radiotherapy treatment one day. He could not face it anymore. It was a difficult time for all of the family.

While I was shocked and upset by the situation, and the stark realisation of mortality — I also experienced it as a time of transition. To this point my parents had been the strong ones — the carers. It felt very much like it was now my turn to assume the role of the strong one, the carer, while Dad was ill. I don't recall experiencing doubt or resentment — it just seemed like the right thing to do at a difficult time. In the words of the singer-songwriter John Mellencamp — 'There is nothing more sad or beautiful than generations changing hands.'

I was fortunate at that time to have a housemate who was studying psychology, and developing a specialisation in crisis counselling. He was an excellent sounding board, and a great friend. I discussed Dad's situation with him, and we identified a psychologist who could help him. I approached the topic gently with Dad — he was very wary of any medical treatment, and did not, I think, have the awareness at that time that he was experiencing psychological trauma. I floated the idea and left it for Dad to consider. He agreed to meet the psychologist and to have an initial discussion. He did this on his own as I recall, but with Mum's support.

I am proud of the way in which Dad embraced counselling, which was explained to him as a simple kit of tools for Dad to use when faced with stressful situations. He has grown enormously as a person as a result, and we have grown far closer as father and son. Dad has continued to develop himself, to read, to meditate, and to share his experiences and learn from others.

Mum passed away in 2011. It was extraordinarily sad, but the way in which Dad approached this stressful time, and this fundamental change in his life, was nothing short of inspiring. About a month after Mum passed away, I asked Dad how he was going. He said to me 'I'm living in the moment. So many friends are asking me to meet them, to have dinner, to catch up — I've just decided I am going to say *yes* to them all.'

Gerry

I was diagnosed in 1998 and had a radical prostatectomy. My first concern was am I going to survive any treatment? I had a suspicion about my heart, so I went through the process of being diagnosed with a heart condition then an angiogram then angioplasty. So I had to recover from that first. I didn't know until a few weeks before the surgery what I was going to do. It was an uncertain time; there was lots of talk of new therapies coming out from some of the centres in the Unites States, so it was confusing and a time of great turmoil. Slowly but surely I came to realise that I needed to understand an awful lot more, really understand how good these statistics actually were compared to what they were saying, there was always more to it than the statistics led you to believe.

Then, when I was in Sydney visiting my granddaughters, I was on the train and there was a sign about a prostate cancer support group there. Believe it or not at that time I had not even checked to see if there was one in Queensland where I live. So I gave them a ring and they were a really good mob! Three guys — one had had radiation, one surgery and one guy was on watchful waiting. They spent an afternoon with me and it was wonderful. I figured out from that conversation what I needed to know about most and how I could find out more.

During the five months which had passed since diagnosis my PSA had gone up from 6.5 to 11 — clearly something had to be done. By the time I had made up my mind about treatment, I thought: 'Well I am stuck with whatever the outcome so I had better get on with it!' I had made up my mind that whatever the outcome of treatment was, I was going to live with it, and accept it and go on from there.

My approach after treatment was to work out what strategies I could apply to make things easier to get over. What I didn't do, and what I should have done, was set myself a goal. Coming up to the end of my accrued sick leave after two months, I decided I had better go back to work. At that time I was still on a couple of pads a day and once I paid attention to this with my exercises very soon I was dry. If I had set myself a goal earlier I would have reached that point sooner. I had decided I wasn't going to get uptight about it no matter what and so I had let this slide. I was just a lazy boy!

Fourteen years on now I guess the main thing that I worry about is my PSA tests. There is always that chance that my PSA will effect a sudden change, but at my age we are looking at death from other causes so you need to keep it in perspective. My main message to men now is when you have a problem to solve you are really looking at making a decision. You have to decide if you are going to act, and then if yes, choose your approach. Make sure that you understand the problem, and break it down into steps. You've got to consider what's important and what needs to be dealt with first, and consider carefully why that's important as against the other things in life that are important to you.

Graham

I was initially diagnosed by my GP in 2009, and had a radical prostatectomy. All I wanted was to have the cancer removed, just get rid of it. It was all very matter of fact at the time, one minute I had a prostate and the next I didn't. My surgeon did actually say to me one day when we were talking: 'We are removing that many prostates at the moment that it is just like picking pineapples.'

I knew of absolutely nobody else who had had their prostate out, so I was totally alone, I didn't know where I could go to for support.

My major problem after surgery was urinary incontinence. I was told that some men suffer from some form of incontinence after a radical prostatectomy, but mine was just terrible. A few days after the operation and prior to leaving the hospital a physiotherapist told me about pelvic floor exercises, which I didn't even know existed until then. Then as I left hospital, I was handed some pads and that was it. I had very little knowledge about incontinence and now I look back I don't know that I researched it enough. I guess I expected the doctor to sort it all out for me.

For two years I struggled with the incontinence, saw three physiotherapists but the best I got down to was five pads a day. Everywhere I went I had to take pads, even on a trip to Turkey! My wife was fabulous about it, she would say: 'It's only wee.' But it's not the fact that it's only wee, it's the fact that you are wet all the time and your skin is wrinkly and you can't get dry, it's just so demoralising. In retrospect I think that it made me a bit aggressive. I would get really angry at other people for complaining about things they should be grateful for. I was thinking: 'Why was it me that had this?' I have never been a person that was a 'why me' type, but it certainly made me one at the time.

Then through a support group I learnt about a surgical treatment for this problem — a sling and it worked! It is absolutely amazing — in hospital overnight and now completely dry!

I decided to also get a penile implant to get over the erectile problems I was experiencing. I had tried everything for this. I tried the tablets and they gave me headaches, and I found the injections didn't suit me either. I am a bit funny with needles, so to decide I was going to have sex then take time out and inject myself and come back — that just wasn't for me.

Honestly, once I got the implant and the sling my whole mindset completely changed. I told the doctor that did the implant that I remember as a young fellow my dad would say that you really feel good if you have a few beers in the fridge but you don't have to go and drink it; and another friend says I am always comfortable if I have chocolate in the fridge. These are the two things that stay in my mind with the implant. You mightn't use it for a week or two but you feel bloody good that you can access it.

It's a mindset thing and you don't understand a lot of this until after the event. You cope, and then you think how did I get through that? But you just do. My mind ticks over all the time about it, but once you are fixed you get much more relaxed about it all. I am almost proud now that I have an implant and a sling.

I know many men may not experience the problems that I experienced, but whatever problems they do experience my message is: 'Don't give up, there is an answer.' I am happy to say I had wonderful support from my wife and friends. Men tend not to talk about their health issues. I have learnt to be more open. If someone is available to listen or help — take the opportunity!

■■■■

Grace Under Fire

In his classic book, *The Old Man and the Sea*, Ernest Hemingway famously said that 'the definition of courage is grace under fire'. Whenever I read this quote I always think of all the men and women I have seen face cancer, taking what is thrown at them, and enduring. This takes courage, every day. Not only do people endure and move step by step and purposefully through this illness experience, they also often find new meaning in their social connections, their relationships and the world around them, take on new challenges in life, and sometimes develop a new way of being in the world.

Many people do say after cancer that although they would not wish this experience on anyone, least of all themselves, they have found benefits in their lives as a result. They also talk about the 'goal posts shifting', where what matters to them now is somewhat different and that their priorities have changed. The experience of cancer can be life altering in ways other than the physical, and for some can produce positive outcomes in unexpected ways.

Searching for Meaning

The 'why me' and wondering how it is that you or your partner came to be facing prostate cancer is a pretty common response to being in this situation. Cancer is not fair, it strikes people from all walks of life and backgrounds, and living a healthy, pure and honest life does not make you bullet proof. A threat to life can lead you to wonder about the meaning of life, and if 'this is it'. People sometimes ask themselves: 'What sort of person do I want to be? What sort of relationships do I want with others, and what do I want my life to be about?'

There are many philosophical traditions, Western and Eastern, that deal with this question: 'What is the meaning of life and what is the meaning of *my* life?' Some people find their religious or spiritual faith helpful and others find reflection, self-questioning and the seeking of knowledge an approach that leads to acceptance and strength. This is a personal and very individual path to walk, and there is no one right way to consider what having had cancer or loving someone who has had cancer, means to you. It is your journey.

It is important to note that some people do not see their diagnosis as a life changing experience. For them, cancer is just another hurdle in life to manage and over-come as soon as they can with the resources they have available. For many others, the cancer experience leads them to revaluate how they view themselves and the world around them. These are the people who often report positive life changes after struggling with their cancer and treatment.

Finding the Good

If the goal posts shifted for you after you found out the diagnosis of prostate cancer, you may have found that some aspects of your life have changed in a positive way. This is often called 'benefit-finding' which is pretty self-explanatory, or 'post-traumatic growth' which is a little more obscure. Both of these terms refer to when a traumatic event, such as a cancer diagnosis, shakes a person's world up to the point that they find themselves re-evaluating their life direction, personal priorities, relationships and future goals. This is an introspective and reflective process that can lead to a sense of personal growth, and for some people decisions to change aspects of their lives. Post-traumatic growth is not confined to the experience of cancer, it can include the experience of war, loss of a loved one, road trauma or accidents. Any trauma where a person has experienced high levels of emotional distress and a threat to either their own well-being or a threat to the well-being of people close to them can lead to personal growth. Post-traumatic growth is its own universe in the sense that this positive aspect of change appears to be a separate outcome to the negative. The positive and negative don't cancel each other out, they co-exist.

A common way post-traumatic growth is expressed by people affected by cancer is that they now pay more care and attention to their loves one and important personal relationships. Alternatively, sometimes a person might find their cancer is the tipping point that leads them to break off a relationship that perhaps has not been right for them for some time. Other people find they develop a new and deeper level of compassion for others and might take up volunteer work for a good cause or try and help others whenever they can. This compassion includes where a person finds within them forgiveness and kindness towards themselves, as well as towards others.

The courage or daring to try new challenges is another way people experience post-traumatic growth. Think of the people you know who have had cancer who take up marathon runs, walks or cycle trips to raise funds for cancer research as well as to challenge themselves physically. Dragon boating, mountain climbing, motorcycle riding, the list goes on. Many of the men and women who contributed their personal experiences about prostate cancer to this book have found their lives changed in these ways after cancer, and even just being prepared to share your story in this way is an act of courage.

Another way that people diagnosed with cancer or their loved ones express post-traumatic growth is reporting a newfound sense of personal strength. This fits with that old saying 'what doesn't kill you, only makes you stronger'. Often people will comment that it wasn't until they were pushed did they realise how much they could deal with. Realising that you can cope with cancer may help you realise that you can cope with any of the challenges that life throws at you.

People who have been diagnosed with cancer often report that their priorities have now shifted. We can all become bogged down in the routine of life — work, paying the bills, commuting. Sometimes it takes something big to awaken us to all the possibilities that life has to offer. After struggling with cancer, some people may decide to spend more time with family and friends and less time at work, and some may decide to pursue life-long dreams that had previously been put on hold. This does not mean that everyone has or even needs to have this type of reaction to their cancer. Just getting through treatment and back to your usual life can be challenge enough.

Rebuilding Your Identity

After prostate cancer, who exactly are you? A person who has had prostate cancer or who loves someone who does? A cancer victim? A cancer survivor? A cancer patient?

Part of recovery is being comfortable with yourself, just as you are, at each stage of your recovery or role as a carer; and for men being okay with the parts of you that may have changed physically. For men who have had prostate cancer the effects of treatment challenge sexual confidence in a way that hits to the core. This can be shattering to your masculinity and view of yourself as a man. Many men have told me rebuilding the masculine and sexual part of themselves is an ongoing 'work in progress'. As well, finding out you have cancer makes it hard to keep acting as if you are invincible, which is a typical 'blokey' attitude to the world and their health in particular. Feeling vulnerable about your health as well as your masculinity in this way is a tough road. Knowing that you are not alone helps. Talking about how this feels either to your partner or to other men who have also experienced prostate cancer can help you work this through to find a sense of coherence and rebuild your confidence.

After being diagnosed with cancer, some people are thrust into positions of role models in their circle of friends and their community. Others willingly take up raising awareness and funds for cancer research and offering support to others. Being diagnosed with cancer can open up a new network of friends, activities and events, and a new identity based on being a cancer survivor. Joining community groups and even taking part in research are just some of the ways that people feel like they can contribute and give back, as well as gain a sense of belonging with others who understand.

I know many people who proudly, and often, will say 'I am cancer survivor', and for them this means being strong, resilient and fearless. Others feel that they do not want to define themselves by their cancer, and see it more as an experience they have moved past. Again, neither way is right or wrong. What is important is to feel strong and confident about yourself and who you are now.

If you have faced the tiger, you know what it means to journey through struggle and difficulty, and this journey belongs to you.

Personal Stories

Below is a personal story from Peter about challenges he took on after his prostate cancer and how this has influenced his life.

Peter

As I talked about earlier (Chapter 2) the diagnosis, treatment and side effects of a radical prostatectomy in 1996 at age 52, left me reeling and searching for answers. My life suddenly deteriorated from being a healthy, fit, in-control, positive individual to one that was desperate, experiencing certain body-symptoms out of control, seriously depressed, bordering on suicidal and harbouring an exceedingly dark, repressed view of the world and the future.

Once I'd made up my mind that I was not going to give up on myself, I reasoned I would need to understand the process I was going through. This was achieved in several ways.

Firstly, gaining the assistance and support of other men who were travelling the same road was imperative.

At this level, we shared personal information and knowledge, developing strength as we empathised with each other. This was reinforced by attending lectures from health professionals of all disciplines involved with cancer and its side effects. Plus reading, studying, talking and asking — it was a time for coming out of 'our cave', regrouping and approaching the fight with this enemy as you would any battle.

As males, our lives have generally been programmed on autopilot, fulfilling stereotypes and traditional agenda roles placed on us by society. For the most part, we didn't mind or have any need to question this — the system worked well, allowing us to gain what we thought was high satisfaction out of life.

Until suddenly, something breaks down, and our expectations of life can't be fulfilled. It is particularly traumatic for men if the breakdown compromises our ability to work, to provide for ourselves and our family and to have sex. (Prostate cancer can jeopardise all of these). At a time like this, it is important to contemplate some universal truths. What is a male? What is sex and how important is it really? And the deeper ones: What is life? Is there a purpose to it? Relationships? God? Happiness? ... the list of unanswered questions goes on ...

This process of readjustment takes time. It is really a search for a new reality — to work out how to redefine yourself, to rebuild a new self-image.

As tough as it seems, illness can provide us with the capacity to gain some new insights and wisdom, to cut through the nonsense and sham. There is no one answer to allow us to achieve this. Everybody will have different strategies to cope with their losses. Basically cancer enables us to think about what's important and to prioritise things in our life. Seven years after my diagnosis and treatment, I felt the need for a sense of closure, to celebrate my new life. I was now nimble again and had developed purpose. I would climb Mt. Kilimanjaro — at almost 6,000m, the African continent's highest peak.

Why climb a mountain to prove anything? Most people would consider the exercise to be irrational. Perhaps, on one level, I see some symbolism of the uphill climb cancer survivors must face and overcome. On another level, it was a chance to measure myself, to balance the depressing threat to my life from cancer with elation for living. After a 60km climb through tropical jungle, hot, stifling but beautiful rainforest, to moorlands, alpine desert and finally, glaciers, ice and snow in sub-zero temperatures, I reached the summit on St. Valentine's Day, 2003.

This was a triumph and satisfied me for some years. However, I had now learned to appreciate life from a larger perspective. Life on earth started 3.8 billion years ago — I had been given one sliver of it to savour. I would live it passionately — I would climb another mountain, higher than Kilimanjaro. In December 2009, at age 66, I began climbing Mt. Aconcagua. At 6959m, the highest peak outside the Himalayas, Aconcagua soars out of the Andes in Argentina.

After eight days, we became trapped by a blizzard fifteen hundred metres below the summit. We were three weeks into the climbing season which had been marked by terrible storms. In that time, of 70 climbers who had attempted the summit, only 5 had succeeded, one of them perishing on the day before our group started for the top.

This news was highly distressing, adding to my fears. At this stage, I was seriously exhausted. I hadn't expected the continuing freezing conditions — minus 30 degrees — and was having trouble sleeping. My hands had been slashed by lifting sharp-edged rocks to keep our tents stable in the high winds, creating difficulty holding utensils to feed and look after myself.

While here, I was subject to an interesting phenomenon. We were advised not to go outside at night to urinate; it was too cold. The correct technique is to kneel inside the tent and deftly pee into a container. I didn't feel confident of achieving this, so I braved the elements outside. Expecting the scene to be black, I was shocked to see the landscape flooded with a burning silver light. The stars and moon were so close and unhindered by atmosphere, they totally blazed. The Southern Cross was on fire right above me. In an intense physical and emotional experience, amounting to an epiphany, I was overwhelmed by a sudden and pleasing awareness that I was in union with the universe. I could reach out and touch the stars and their trillions of atoms would be the same as mine. The feeling of inclusion has never left me.

The next day, our guide told us we would die if we tried for the summit, so we chose life and headed back. There was some disappointment, but to me, there was a deeper satisfaction — that of knowing I had challenged myself and had decided my own fate. The journey was much more than summiting and conquering a mountain. The ultimate journey was to within and to conquer oneself.

Appendix

This is a brief list of places to you might wish to start for more detailed information on specific issues. For medical or treatment questions your doctor is the best first point of call for advice that is personalised to your situation. Contact details were accurate at time of printing.

Helpful Publications

Sex and Sexuality

Saving Your Sex Life: A Guide for Men with Prostate Cancer. John P. Mulhall, Hilton Publishing, Bethesda, MD, 2010. ISBN 9780980064964.

After Prostate Cancer: A What-comes-next guide to a safe and informed recovery. Arnold Melman, MD & Rosemary E. Newnham. New York: Oxford University Press, 2011. ISBN 9780195399660.

A gay man's guide to prostate cancer: Gerald Perlman and Jack Drescher, Haworth Medical Press, United States, ISBN 9781560235521.

Urinary Problems

Conquering Incontinence: A New and Physical Approach to a Freer Lifestyle Exercise. Peter Dornan, Allen & Unwin, Australia 2003. ISBN 9781741141443.

Mindfulness and Mediation

Happy For No Good Reason: A meditators guide by Shankarananda, Swami, Motilal Banasidass, India, 2004 ISBN 9788120820050.

Full Catastrophe Living: Using the Wisdom of Your Body and Mind to Face Stress, Pain, and Illness Jon Kabat-Zin. Delta Publishing, 1990 ISBN 9780385303125.

Prostate Cancer Treatments

Localised Prostate Cancer: A guide for men and their families 4th Ed, the Australian Prostate Cancer Collaboration, Australia 2010. ISBN 0957993811, electronic copies are available from Prostate Cancer Foundation of Australia http://www.prostate.org.au/articleLive/pages/Download-Information.html or hardcopies can be ordered by calling 1800 22 00 99.

Advanced Prostate Cancer: A guide for men and their families, Cancer Council Australia, 2009 ISBN 9780980742107. Electronic copies are available from Cancer Council Australia http://www.cancer.org.au/Healthprofessionals/clinicalguidelines/prostatecancer.htm or hardcopies can be ordered by calling 131120.

Complementary Medicine

Promoting Wellness for Prostate Cancer Patients, Mark A Moyad, Ann Arbor Editions US 2010, ISBN 9781930842045.

Wellbeing

Taking Care of yourself and your family: A resource book for good mental health. John Ashfield, Peacock Publications, Australia, ISBN 1921008490. Available free in Australia from *Beyondblue* by calling 1300 22 4636.

What Women (and Their Men) Need to Know About Prostate Cancer. Irena Madjar in collaboration with Gail Tingle. Health Research Association, 2007, ISBN 0646468529, 9780646468525.

Exercise

Exercise and Sports Science Australia (ESSA) — www.essa.org.au provide details of registered exercise professionals with University qualifications who are able to conduct exercise training with people who have had cancer or other chronic illnesses. The ESSA website has a section in their main page on How to Find an Exercise Physiologist: www.essa.org.au.

American College of Sports Medicine (ACSM — www.acsm.org) provides a similar service as does the British Association of Sport and Exercise Sciences, BASES — www.bases.org.uk/ in the United Kingdom.

Cancer Helplines and Support Groups

Australia

Prostate cancer support groups: To contact a prostate cancer support group in your local area look up Prostate Cancer Foundation of Australia website (http://www.prostate. org.au/articleLive/pages/Support-Groups.html) or call Freecall: 1800 220 099. Prostate Cancer Foundation of Australia is the peak national body for prostate cancer in Australia dedicated to reducing the impact of prostate cancer on Australian men, their partners, families and the wider community through research, awareness and support.

Cancer Council Helpline is a free, confidential telephone information and support service run by Cancer Councils in each state and territory in Australia. Specially trained staff are available to answer questions about cancer and provide support. Call 13 11 20 (local call cost from anywhere in Australia but mobile calls charged at mobile rates), open between 9am and 5pm, Monday to Friday, however some states have extended hours.

North America

The Us Too International Prostate Cancer Education and Support Network is a nonprofit, grassroots organisation that provides support for prostate cancer patients, survivors, their spouses and partners and families. More details can be found on their website http://www.ustoo.org/. They have a toll free line to link for patients and concerned others to resources regarding diagnosis, treatment options and support systems and phone support from a prostate cancer survivor. Call 1-800-80-UsTOO (1-800-808-7866), M-F 9am-5pm Central Time.

United Kingdom

The Prostate Cancer Support Federation can connect you to a support group through their National Help Line on 0845 601 0766. The web address for this group is http://prostatecancerfederation.org.uk/index.htm.

Other Useful Websites

http://blog.renewintimacy.org/
The Center for Intimacy after Cancer Therapy, Inc., is n nonprofit organization dedicated to helping couples renew their intimacy after cancer. Founders and Co-Executive Directors: Ralph and Barbara Alterowitz.

http://www.prostate.org.au/

Prostate Cancer Foundation of Australia is the peak national body for prostate cancer in Australia. We are dedicated to reducing the impact of prostate cancer on Australian men, their partners, families and the wider community through research, awareness and support.

http://www.prostatehealth.org.au/

The Lions Australian Prostate Cancer Website was developed by the education committee of The Australian Prostate Cancer Collaboration (APCC) with funding from the Lions International Clubs of Australia to assist men affected by prostate cancer and their families.

http://prostatenet.com/page/

The Prostate Net is an international organization that uses a matrix of informational techniques (Web site, 800#, email and personal team counselors, public forums, newsletters and community disease interventions) to address disease risk awareness and early disease interdiction.

CPSIA information can be obtained
at www.ICGtesting.com
Printed in the USA
LVOW04s0805150516
488307LV00009B/171/P